Beautiful
BIRTH

Practical techniques to help
you enjoy your birth

T0145934

SUZANNE YATES

pinter
&
martin

'…a useful "go to" book for massage, visualisation, birth positions,
simple shiatsu and exercises for labour.'
Alice Lyon, community midwife for 25 years

'…encourages a man to seek out opportunities to connect deeply with his pregnant partner…'
Mark Harris, author of *Men, Love & Birth*

'…gives couples some tools to use during birth together, bringing them
strength as a team and creating a sense of confidence. I love it!'
Beccy Hands, massage therapist and owner of the Mother Box

First published in 2008 in the United Kingdom by Carroll & Brown Publishers Limited

This edition published by Pinter & Martin 2017, reprinted 2018, 2024

Managing Art Editor Emily Cook

Photograper Jules Selmes

Text © Suzanne Yates 2008, 2017

A CIP catalogue record for this book is available from
the British Library.

ISBN 978-1-78066-450-7

Pinter & Martin Ltd
Unit 803 Omega Works
4 Roach Road
London E3 2PH

www.pinterandmartin.com

Contents

Foreword

The use of massage and touch in labour can improve your experiences of birth. In this second edition of *Beautiful Birth*, Suzanne enlightens both prospective parents and birth professionals about a holistic, body and mind approach to pregnancy and preparing for birth. Pinter & Martin, her new publishers, aptly recognise her knowledgeable and clear approach to birth preparation, including useful perspectives of massage, more expanded information on shiatsu, breathing techniques and new updated visualisations. This lovely book is a hands-on guide, supporting your individual voyage through labour by promoting a relaxed mind, encouraging practical touch techniques and promotes a powerful sense of togetherness between you, your baby and your partner.

I am a practicing midwife, private massage therapist and co-director of a charity and social enterprise, The Birth & Wellbeing Partnership, which provides massage and counselling for those needing this combined approach through pregnancy, birth and new parenthood. I therefore see the need for this effective, holistic support daily.

It was my love of Suzanne's multifaceted approach to bodywork that inspired me to join her pregnancy massage course, not long after my son was born, in 2006. Suzanne's work encourages thoughtful communication between you and your partner. In fact, the inspiration sparked during Suzanne's courses motivated me to begin my journey in becoming and being a midwife. A massaging midwife.

My own philosophy is that the use of relaxation, massage and touch promotes **Calm**, **Comfort** and **Connection**, the themes explored in my midwifery dissertation 'How can the use of massage can improve women's experiences of labour and birth?'. However, these themes can be incorporated into your birth preparation in diverse ways, as Suzanne clarifies with the addition of utilising positions that promote comfort and progress, different visualisations and breathing techniques for example. After all, the important aspect is to find a technique that suits you.

Calm: Massage and positive touch encourages you to relax, promotes your oxytocin (the significant hormone that fosters love, supports labour and breastfeeding), reduces anxiety and deepens slower, parasympathetic responses. This physical aspect of wellbeing is complimented by Suzanne's relaxation and visualisation chapters beautifully.

Comfort: A focused and intentional touch improves your experiences of pain by distracting your brain from such strong sensations, promoting an abundance of your natural pain relieving hormones such as endorphins and reducing the impact of psychological aspects of pain linked to your own personal, cultural and social experiences. What works especially well in this book is the explanation of techniques you can use in many positions, promoting active and upright movement that encourages your natural birth processes, whilst inspiring your instinctive response to your baby's position and the best way for you to be, and cope well.

Connection: Improving the quality of support you receive and the sense of togetherness that touch and massage techniques provides, improves relationships between you, your baby and your partner, particularly when practiced regularly in pregnancy. Communication is enhanced, an important aspect of birth support. I love the images Suzanne has chosen to illustrate this, especially in the labour chapter.

Interestingly, it has also been recognised that if you use massage and touch in pregnancy, you are more likely to use massage on your baby after birth. Suzanne gives some simple tips to continue massaging your baby after birth. We now know that this has an enormous impact on both yours and your baby's mental health; by promoting attachment, stimulating your baby's sensory development, prompting appetite and growth. Your babies brain development responds to this wonderful connection and is crucial for their long-term wellbeing.

Although this book is aimed at promoting a physiological birth, where possible, Suzanne's techniques are adaptable and useful in many ways; and she outlines their use in situations such as supporting you should your birth be induced, as preparation for your elective caesarean, keeping a continuity of calm when circumstances or environments change and in establishing breastfeeding. Suzanne's thoughtful, practical approach will provide you and your partner with skills not just for your pregnancy, but for family life in general; any time of stress or struggle will benefit from these techniques.

I highly recommend this book as an integral and important part of your wellbeing in this time of physical, psychological and emotional change. Practise these tools and techniques regularly so that they feel comfortable and easy. This will encourage relaxed familiarity, prompting beautiful pregnancy and birth experiences. These are practical skills you can learn now but will go on to love for years to come.

Claire Nutt, autumn 2017
@MassageMidwife

Your birth journey

Congratulations. A special day is nearing – your baby's birth – and my aim in writing this book is to help make that day one of joy and celebration.

This book is about helping you learn how to work with your body and your baby so that you can enjoy your experience of the birth as much as possible. A key element is using the power of touch and massage, and the physical and emotional connection between you and your birth partner. I hope you find it inspiring and fun to use and that it enhances your birth experience. Even if the process is not as enjoyable as you hoped, by learning to work with your body and your baby, you still can feel you gave your best whatever happens.

In our culture, preparation for birth is often needlessly marked by fear and anxiety. We ask ourselves if we can cope with the pain. But birth is about much more than physical pain. It is an exciting journey into places in your body and mind and your relationship with your partner to which you have never been before. It is a journey in which you will learn more about yourself than you ever thought possible.

Preparation

If you have never had a baby before, preparing for the birth can be strange because so much is unknown. You don't know exactly what it will be like, how long it will take, when it will start or how hard it is going to be.

Because your attitude will influence your journey, you need to prepare your mind as well as your body: If you expect it to be hard, you risk making it so by becoming tense and anxious; but if you expect it to be a positive experience, and prepare well by learning how to relax your body and mind, then it is more likely to be enjoyable. Even if you have a "difficult" birth, by approaching it with a positive attitude you will be better able to handle any problems that may arise.

Visualizations and breathing exercises are useful ways of preparing yourself mentally, and you will find plenty of them in this book. They can help you to achieve mental relaxation, which is important to both the emotional and physical aspects of giving birth. The connection between a relaxed mind and physical ability is well known in the sporting world; in switching off our minds and feeling what we are doing, it can become easier to master, for example, the ski slope or the surf, and the same principle applies to birth. Ultimately you need to be able to get past your conscious mind so that you can tap into more instinctive aspects.

A natural process

It's important to remember that giving birth is a natural process with which women's bodies are designed to cope. This simple fact is often forgotten in our technological age, when all discomfort and physical pain is seen as bad and something to be numbed. Although we tend to associate pain with suffering, the two aren't always connected. While toothache, for example, is telling you that something is wrong with your body, the pain of labour has a different purpose. It helps you to be more aware of what your body and mind needs to do during birth. If, for instance, you are in the wrong position, it is helpful to feel discomfort so that you can change it. It is also helpful for you to feel the pressure of the baby as he or she journeys down the birth canal, so that you can respond to his or her needs.

Most mothers, if they are prepared and well supported, find that they don't need drugs to help them through childbirth. The pain is usually not so overwhelming and, as you shall see, there are many natural ways of relieving it. Our bodies do sometimes need additional help, however, and today we are fortunate in that we have access to pain-killing drugs and medical interventions if we need them. Both have their place, but they are too often seen as the first way to approach birth, not the last. The majority of mothers can manage childbirth by tapping into their own resources and, when they give birth in this way, they feel they have discovered a wonderful power and strength within themselves. Helping you achieve that power and strength is my reason for writing this book.

Suzanne Yates

How to use this book

You and your partner are about to embark on an incredible journey. Rather than impose a "one size fits all" itinerary, my aim is to help you find the right emotional and physical approach..

As an expectant mother, you know the most about yourself and your unborn baby; how you find your way through birth lies within your own body and awareness. You are the person who is most likely to be able to notice if things are going well, or if there is a problem. You are the one who has to decide what kind of external support you may need.

This book is intended primarily as a practical guide to lots of useful exercises that can help you engage with your birth journey. Think of it as a toolbox from which you can pick and choose "tools" that can help you achieve a more aware and less painful birth.

The first part describes and explains how to use the main practical tools of breathing/ visualization, physical preparation and massage. As well as explaining how to practise the techniques, I also include information on when and why they are useful in labour, and if any variations might be needed.

The second part guides you through labour, explaining its stages, helping you to understand how you respond to pain and the unknown, enabling you to ready your birth space and partner, and preparing your baby for the birth. I suggest that you read the whole book from start to finish and then go back and practise the

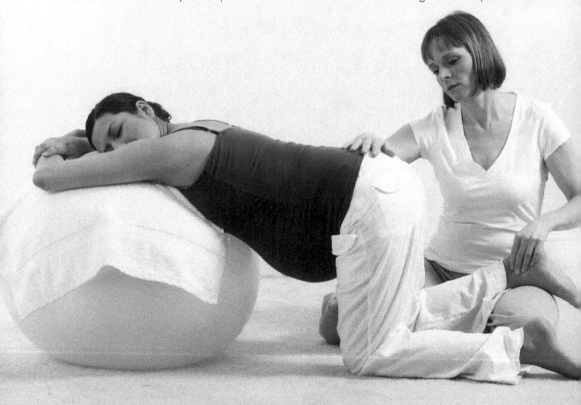

exercises that most appeal to you. You don't have to use everything in this book in order to benefit from it. You may just want to read it through to stimulate your own ideas or to identify the type of birth preparation class that feels best for you. You can then use the book to reinforce what you learn in class. Like your body and your baby, this is your book; use it in whichever way works best for you. If you are unsure about anything, please seek further advice from a relevant health professional.

A word about partners

Throughout I have referred to the birth partner as "he" to save awkwardness when writing. Though many women will be working with their babies' fathers, you may choose a female birth partner – a companion, friend or relative or even a practitioner trained in my "Well Mother" techniques. The techniques are suitable for working with both sexes; just read "he" as "she"!

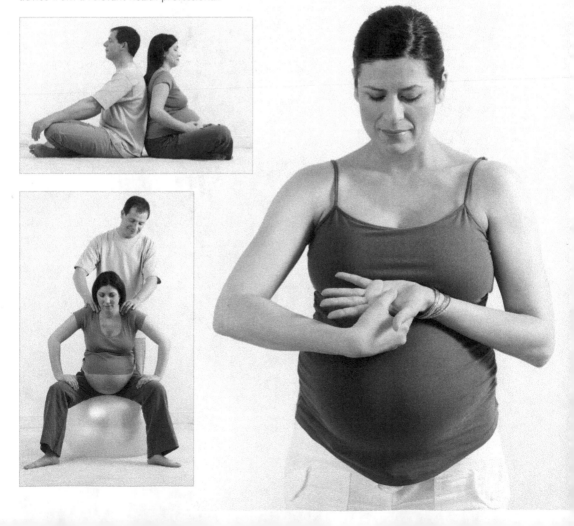

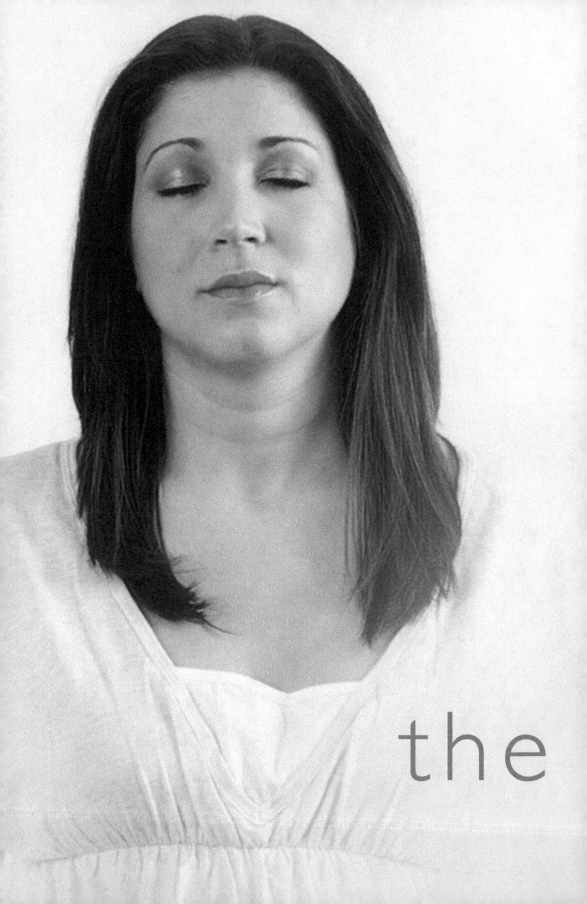

the

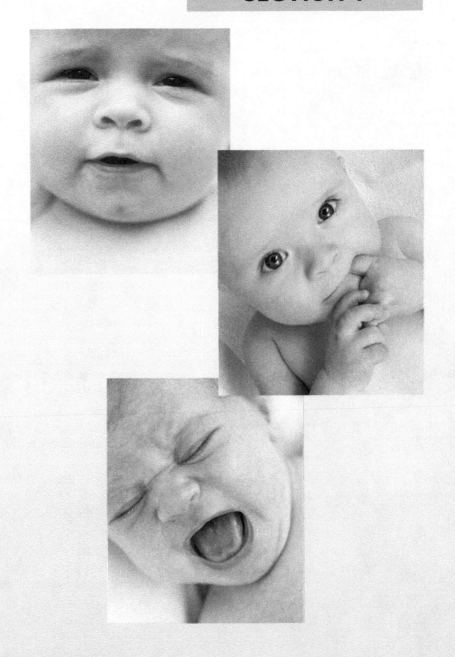

fundamentals

Before you begin...

The activities in this book are designed to help you prepare for childbirth, something that you should begin to focus on during your last trimester. Most of the exercises, visualizations and massage routines can be practised from 28 weeks of pregnancy; there are just a few things that are more suitable for just before the birth or during labour itself. As listening to your body and your baby is central to the process, it is best if you decide exactly when each activity feels appropriate for you. Not all of the work is going to feel right for everyone at all times.

If at any point you don't feel comfortable doing something – whether it is breathing, an exercise or some massage – then don't carry on with it. Your body changes daily in pregnancy, and it can be that on some days you will feel like practising certain things and on other days you won't. So do try things more than once if you don't immediately take to them, because you may find that one day something you didn't like before now feels right. This in itself is good practice for labour as during labour how you feel will change frequently and you will have to adapt your response to the changes.

FINDING THE TIME AND SPACE

You should set aside some time each day, even if it is only a few minutes, for you and your partner to tune in to your baby and your breathing. What you can accomplish depends a lot on how long it is until the birth and how much time you can devote to the activities.

If you only have a couple of weeks to go, try and set aside at least a half an hour each day. If you have longer until the birth, you might want to aim for one 30-minute session per week, and other daily sessions of 5–10 minutes. If you already have children, you might want to include them in your preparation. They often find many of the exercises fun.

It is helpful to have a comfortable space in which to practise the exercises. Ideally, you want somewhere quiet where you can focus without distractions or interruptions. Make sure the space is warm enough for you, because if you feel cold, you won't be able to relax. As a lot of the work is done on the floor, it is best if the space is carpeted. If it has a bare wooden floor, put a rug or yoga mat down and work on that.

Have some cushions or pillows available to make yourself more comfortable when resting in different positions. If you have bought a pillow for breastfeeding, you could start using that now for relaxation. Many mothers find that they like using a gym ball as it is great for sitting or leaning on; others prefer a beanbag to rest on.

To make your space more comfortable and relaxing, you might like to have music playing and/or to burn a scented candle. You can choose to have some nice objects around such as inspiring or relaxing photos or pictures, or objects that hold a special meaning for you or you might prefer to have a clear space or even to work outdoors.

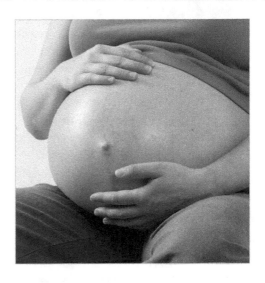

Creating a comfortable space to work in will also help you to identify environments you find supportive. This will be useful when you are planning your birthing space, especially if you are going to have a home birth. If you intend to be in hospital when you go into labour,, however, you can use this knowledge to choose items to have with you that can help re-create some aspects of your home environment.

Use whatever is useful to you,
whenever it is useful for you.
Listen to your body and to your baby.

Breathing and visualization

Breath is fundamental to life. By breathing deeply, you are ensuring that you and your baby are getting a good supply of oxygen. However, deep breathing is not just about inhaling and exhaling air. It is also a way of taking in and letting go of emotions. With the in breath you can draw in what you need both physically and emotionally while the out breath enables you to let go of things and to relax. With the out breath you can rid yourself not only of old air but also of negative emotions and any tension in your body.

In the past, childbirth classes often emphasized fairly complicated breathing techniques for labour, which had to be learnt from early on in pregnancy. These have largely fallen out of favour because they tend to involve dissociation, a process in which the mother mentally separates herself from what is going on with her body. She does this by using techniques such as counting, or focusing on something outside her body. Aspects of this approach may work for some mothers, but most tend to find the techniques overly complicated and cause them to retreat inside their heads rather than work with their bodies. Pain research carried out with athletes shows that simple techniques involving association – connecting and working with the body, and consciously going through the pain – are the most effective.

The breathing techniques in this book are simpler than those used in the past, but more effective. They include working to deepen the breath, focusing on the out breath, and using sound and visualization. Some are intended for just you to do, but others are for both you and your birth partner. It is important for both partners to practise these, because they will help you to connect with each other.

If you have confidence in your body's ability to give birth easily and safely, you will approach the big event without the worries or fears that can come if that confidence is lacking. One way to boost your confidence is by learning how to listen to your body and to your baby, and how to connect with them in an instinctive way during labour. Your birth partner, whoever he or she may be, can learn to work with you and your baby and also learn specific techniques to support you during labour.

Visualizations are an important part of this book, and will enable you to use your imagination in a focused way. They will help you to switch off your conscious mind and tap into the power of your subconscious. They work best when you combine them with deep breathing, and you should always begin using visualization by focusing on your breath.

Good breathing is also important when you exercise and practise the different birth positions, because it can help you be more relaxed within them. When doing any of the massage techniques you need to be relaxed, and your breathing as well as your position can help you achieve this.

Breathing underpins everything

BASIC DEEP BREATHING

This is an important exercise for both you and your partner to practise. The aim of it is to help you connect with your rhythm of breathing and understand how to deepen it. Then you can use your awareness of this type of deep breathing in all the other breathing exercises.

Beginning the breathing

Begin by finding a comfortable position, such as sitting or lying down, or leaning over a ball or cushions. Either close your eyes, if that feels appropriate, or stare at a nearby object such as a flower, or an image you find inspiring or relaxing, or a candle flame. Now simply focus your mind on following the movement of your breath as you breathe in and out. Become aware of the pattern of your breathing, without altering it in any way. Notice for how long you breathe out and for how long you breathe in; see for how long you can pause between each breath.

Finding a pattern

After a while, just focus on your out breath and allow it to deepen. With each out breath, breathe a little bit more slowly. As you breathe more slowly the breath will lengthen and deepen. See how slowly and deeply you can breathe without forcing the breath.

Now find a simple deep breathing pattern with which you feel comfortable. Take long, slow out breaths, pausing until you need to breathe in again, followed by long, slow in breaths. It is best to breathe in through your nose and out through your mouth.

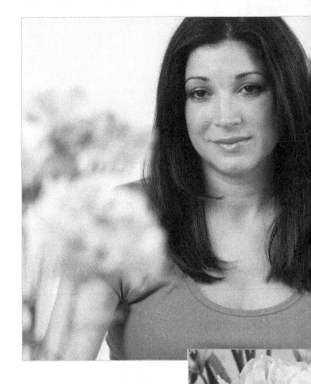

Being aware of your abdominal muscles

As you breathe out, notice if your abdominal muscles are contracting. If they are, emphasize these drawing-in movements when you breathe out and try to expand the muscles when you breathe in,. Do be careful not to force any of these movements.

If your abdominal muscles are pushing out as you breathe out, then try to draw them in, but do this without forcing them. You can rest your hands gently on your abdomen, and draw them towards you with each out breath to try

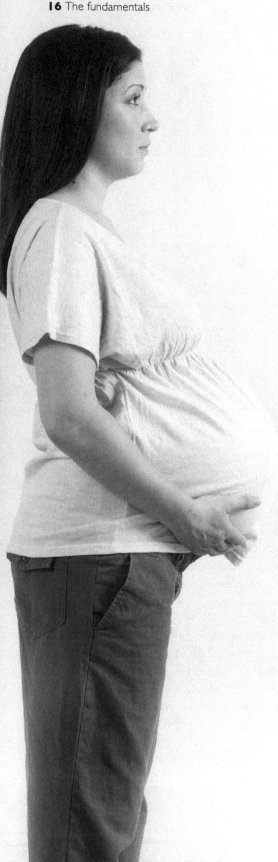

to emphasize this movement. This is the correct way to breathe with your abdominal muscles drawing in when you breathe out.

Now place your hands on your lower abdomen, below your navel, while you focus on your breathing. Feel the rise and fall of your breath, and as you breathe out, feel your muscles contract and gently draw your hands in. As you breathe in, feel your abdomen gently pushing against your hands as the muscles lengthen. This may be a very subtle movement, especially later on in your pregnancy as you start running out of space. Please don't force this movement in any way, just allow it to happen.

Awareness of ribs and spine

Take notice of what is happening to your ribs and spine as you breathe out and in. When you breathe out, your diaphragm rises, your ribcage contracts and your spine softens, but don't slump: keep your spine straight and not curled up or constricted. When you breathe in again, feel how your diaphragm falls, your ribcage expands and your spine extends.

Free movement of your spine will help with the movement of your ribs and diaphragm. As you breathe out, feel your body letting go and gently relaxing from head to toe. As you breathe in and your chest fills with air, feel your spine naturally lengthen, this time with a little more power behind it.

Letting go

As you breathe out through your mouth, let go of your jaw and throat muscles and almost sigh the breath out. Release and relax with each out breath. Then focus on breathing down into your pelvic floor and letting go of any tension in the muscles there. Relaxing your jaw, throat and pelvic floor muscles on the out breath is very helpful during labour. Emphasize this letting go and opening up if you are close to giving birth, but do it more gently if that time is still some way off.

Keep focusing on your breathing in whatever way helps you to breathe in and out deeply and in relaxing fashion. Always concentrate on the out breaths, and simply allow your body to breathe in without making any conscious effort to help it. Notice how deeply and slowly you are breathing now, and how your body is feeling. You can use this breathing with all the visualizations that follow later.

Focus your mind

Now switch your focus to your mind. With each out breath, let go of any distracting thoughts and allow your mind to become more and more deeply relaxed. If you are doing this exercise with your eyes open, focus your thoughts on the object you are looking at. If your eyes are closed, focus on an internal image, for example by imagining your abdomen is like a balloon. As you breathe out, the balloon deflates and your abdomen gets smaller. As you breathe in, the balloon inflates so your abdomen gets larger.

Stay breathing and focusing in whichever way you find most helpful for at least 5 minutes. When you feel you need to ease out of your deep breathing relaxation, with each out breath gradually become more aware of the position in which you are resting, and the room around you, and gradually ease out of your relaxation.

RELAXING BREATH

This is another exercise for both you and your partner. It will show you how to use your breath to release tension from your body, which is an important skill to have during labour.

Beginning the breathing

Sit or lie down comfortably, close your eyes and become aware of the pattern of your breathing without altering it in any way. Notice how long you breathe out for and how long you breathe in for. After a while, just focus on your out breath and allow it to deepen. With each out breath, breathe a little bit more slowly, and as you breathe more slowly, each breath will lengthen and deepen.

Release any tension

As you breathe out, be aware of your whole body. Feel where there are areas of tension and allow them to let go, starting at your head.

Notice how your face is. Are you holding any tension in your cheeks or eyes or jaw? If so, allow some tension to be released as you breathe out, so that with each breath your face becomes more and more deeply relaxed.

Now work your way down through your body, releasing tension in each part of it with a short series of out breaths. Begin with your neck and shoulders, followed by your chest, ribs and the front of your body, and then the back.

Next, turn your attention to your limbs. Soften and relax your arms and hands and allow each hand to open out, like a flower unfurling. Finally, release the tension in your legs and feet. Soften and relax them and let your toes unfurl like a butterfly uncurling.

With each out breath you will feel more and more deeply relaxed. Stay in this experience of deep relaxation for as long as you wish, then when you feel ready to come back out of it, slowly focus on the position of your body. Gradually become more aware of the space around you, feel the space you are resting on and feel the support it is giving. When you are ready, open your eyes.

BABY BREATH HUG

Many mothers find that being actively aware of their babies during labour, rather than fixating on any discomfort or pain, gives them a more positive attitude and makes the experience more bearable if not even enjoyable. The aim of this exercise, which is performed by the mother only, is to help her focus on her baby more readily.

Getting in touch

As you breathe out, place your hands on your lower abdomen and focus on your baby. With each out breath, as you feel your hands being drawn in by the movement of your abdominal muscles, feel that you are gently hugging your baby. You may feel your baby move. As you breathe in, feel that you are creating more space for her. With each out breath, try to be aware of the position of your baby. Can you feel or do you know where her spine is? Can you sense her arms and legs?

If your baby is in a good position, head down and back towards your front, visualize her head gradually going deeper down into your pelvis as she engages in preparation for birth. Be aware of how your baby's time in your womb is gradually coming to an end, and allow yourself to feel comfortable with the thought of letting your baby move out into the world.

If your baby is not in such a good position, either head away from your pelvis, or back against your back, visualize how she might be able to get into a better position. You can talk to her about why she feels comfortable in the position she is in and how, if she moves, her journey out of your body will be easier. You can also talk to your baby about your hopes for the birth and try to tune in to how the birth may be for her.

Now just spend some time relaxing with your baby and enjoy just being with her, aware of whatever thoughts, feelings and sensations you are experiencing. After some time, bring your focus back to the way you are breathing and gradually ease out of your relaxation.

BREATHING TOGETHER

This exercise helps both you and your partner to make an antenatal connection with your baby. This connection also can be useful during labour.

Find a comfortable position in which your partner can settle next to you with one hand on your lower back – wherever it feels most comfortable – and one hand on your abdomen. You could sit with your partner next to you, rest on all fours over a ball, or lie on your side with some cushions placed under your knees, belly or chest.

Connect with your baby

Breathe out slowly and deeply together, using the basic deep breathing technique. As you breathe out and relax, your partner will gradually become more aware of the rhythm of your breathing, and can adjust his to match it. After a while, your partner also can begin to be more aware of the baby beneath his hands. Maybe the baby will make his presence felt as soon as your partner touches you, by kicking or moving around. With each out breath, your partner can focus more on the baby and will feel more connected with both him and you.

You can respond to your baby in whatever way feels appropriate. You could try some gentle stroking over his body, or talk to him, maybe using the name you call him while in the womb or the name you are going to call him when he is born.

When you feel you have a good connection with each other and with your baby, try this exercise in different positions, for example on all fours, sitting, standing, or lying next to each other. In each position notice the pattern of your breathing, how comfortable you are and how your baby is, and spend as long as you want to in each position. If you like, you can add the abdominal massage exercise (see page 67) on to this one.

Making sounds with your breath

A baby's sense of sound develops while he is still in the womb. Singing or listening to songs in pregnancy and then playing the same songs in labour can be very reassuring to him, and after birth he will still respond to the same sounds. Music often uses the rhythm of the heartbeat, as this is the sound that we have all heard for nine months as babies in the womb. This type of rhythmic sound is very soothing for babies, but they appear to get distressed at the sounds of hard rock and harsh, very loud, sudden and un-rhythmical sounds.

Whatever type of music you feel you want during your labour, do make sure that you listen to it regularly during the last few weeks of your pregnancy. That way, it is not only relaxing and familiar to you, but also to your baby.

As well as having music playing during their labour, some mothers like to make lots of sounds with their breathing, while others are quieter and tend to go inside themselves. If you feel that you will want to make sounds, here are some exercises that will help.

AAAH

Begin this exercise with the basic deep breathing technique. With each out breath, become more deeply relaxed. When you feel fully relaxed, clench your jaw and grit your teeth. Observe what happens to your breathing and also what you can feel in your perineum and vaginal area. Now open and relax your jaw and make an "aaah" sound.

Observe again your breathing and what you feel in your perineum and vagina. You should notice that as you relax your jaw and make the sound, you breathe out more deeply and your perineum and vagina relax. By letting go of your jaw as you make the sound, you allow your pelvis to relax. You can achieve this effect with any open throat sound, but those that are most helpful are the "aaah" sounds.

BAAA, PAAA, MAAAAA

There is a chant in Sanskrit, the ancient language of India and one of the oldest, that many mothers find helpful. .

The chant uses the sounds "baaa baaa", "paaa paaa", and "maaaaa". It is interesting that these are labial sounds, which are the first basic sounds that a baby can make using his lips. Another interesting point is that in many languages they form the roots of words for baby (baba), father (papa) and mother (mama).

Repeat the sounds in whichever way you want: say or sing them or play around with them, making them longer or shorter, higher or lower. Feel the sounds in your body and be aware of how your baby is responding to them.

Babies, both in the womb and once they are born, respond well to these particular sounds. Eventually, focus on the rhythm of your breathing and gradually ease yourself out of your relaxation.

VISUALIZATION EXERCISES

Using mental images can help you focus your attention in whatever way works best for you. You can use the following ideas for some of the things covered in section 2, for example, when you want to create your birth space (see page 104), choose your birth partner (see page 108), and prepare your baby for the birth (see page 112). You can play around with these ideas and create any visualization you want.

To do these visualizations, you need to be in the last couple of weeks of your pregnancy – you don't want to start focusing on labour before then. You also will find it helpful to practise them with your birth partner, who can perhaps even read out the scripts to you. That way your partner will get to know what you are going to be doing in labour.

Preparing for labour

This exercise helps you to begin to focus on moving from being pregnant to feeling ready to go into labour. When a mother goes overdue it is often because, on some level, either she or her baby, or both, are not quite ready for labour. Maybe they are scared, or maybe they have enjoyed the pregnancy and subconsciously don't want to move on to the next stage.

Breathe deeply, and when you feel relaxed, begin to be aware of your baby in your womb. Imagine how she is moving down into your pelvis and getting into a good position for

STAGES OF LABOUR

Childbirth is traditionally divided into four stages (more detailed descriptions of the four stages of labour in the chapter starting on page 86).

In Chinese medicine labour is seen as expressions of movement of elements.

First stage
Water: moving from Yin to Yang, like rising waves of water, the contractions become stronger.

Second stage
Wood: with the strong downward movement of the wood energy and its creative power, the baby is born.

Third stage
Movement from wood to fire: wood needed to birth placenta but it changes into fire with joy emerging from the heart to greet the baby.

Fourth stage
Bonding, creating the family. Fire and metal: deepening your heart (fire) connection with your baby but beginning to create new identities in the mother-child relationship (metal).

Earth supports all stages: foundation and regulating the contractions of all stages.

In this safe space, allow yourself to explore any negative feelings you may have about labour

labour. Feel your cervix softening and thinning. Feel your body preparing. How is your body preparing? How is your mind preparing? What are you finding helpful? How are you feeling about the birth? Are you looking forward to it? Are you afraid? Are you feeling ready to let go of your baby and allow her out into the world? Is there anything you feel is blocking you from going into labour?

In this safe space, allow yourself to explore any negative feelings you may have about labour. If you don't feel ready, why don't you feel ready? Explore your feelings until you feel ready to go into labour. Give these feelings space so that you can understand what they are about. When you have understood them, let them go. Now say to yourself, "My body and my baby are ready for labour."

When you feel relaxed and comfortable as you think about labour, focus once more on your breathing and gradually ease back to your body in this moment.

ELEMENTS

The Chinese saw the human body as a microcosm of the universe and developed the movement of the five elements as a way of viewing this. The elements offer a way to connect with different energies in the body, which affect us physically and emotionally. Each element is characterized by a colour or colours; is associated with a particular organ or organs and bodily function; encompasses a human experience; and is represented by a major body component. You can spend time with each element in nature such as sitting alongside a stream or fire and you also can use them in visualizations.

Yin and Yang
Symbol: expressions of the whole
Yin: night, inward, gathering, quiet, space between the contractions
Yang: day, outward, expansive, the contractions
Birth is a movement from Yin to Yang: bringing baby out from the watery space of the womb.
The elements represent a movement from the most Yin: Water to the most Yang: Fire.

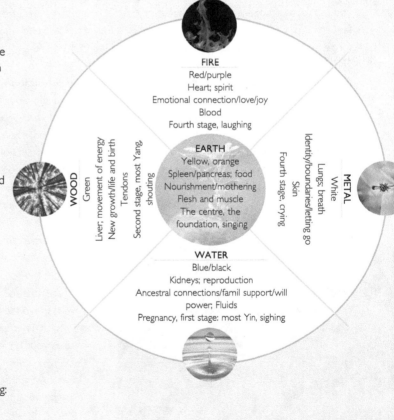

FIRE
Red/purple
Heart; spirit
Emotional connection/love/joy
Blood
Fourth stage, laughing

EARTH
Yellow, orange
Spleen/pancreas; food
Nourishment/mothering
Flesh and muscle
The centre, the foundation, singing

WOOD
Green
Liver; movement of energy
New growth/life and birth
Tendons
Second stage, most Yang, shouting

METAL
White
Lungs; breath
Identity/boundaries/letting go
Skin
Fourth stage, crying

WATER
Blue/black
Kidneys; reproduction
Ancestral connections/famil support/will power; Fluids
Pregnancy, first stage: most Yin, sighing

FIRST STAGE BREATHING

During labour's first stage, you may find that all you need to do is simply focus on the movement of your breath, to breathe out slowly and deeply and to allow the in breath to come into your body. As the contractions get stronger and more intense, continue to focus on your breath, especially the out breath. Simply by doing this, you may find a rhythm that supports the first stage. If that is all you need to do, don't feel that you have to do anything else.

Finding a focus

Some mothers find that they like to use the out breath as a focus for other things. You may find you simply need to relax tense parts of your body as you breathe out. As you breathe out, you can focus on opening up your hands or your feet. You might like to use some of the open throat sounds or simply open and relax your jaw and throat. However, you may find it helpful to focus on an image, a word or a physical object.

At each stage, I have suggested some images to help you to open up and establish a rhythm and connection with each first-stage contraction. Try them to see if any suit you, or if you feel inspired by other images, go with those. Bear in mind that these are only suggestions and it is important you find what is right for you. Your partner might find it helpful to know the

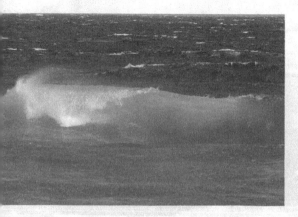

image you are using, so that he can focus on the same thing during the contraction. If you are focusing on a word, then it may be helpful for your partner to speak the word out loud to you during each contraction. If you are focusing on an image, you might find it helpful if your partner talks you through it. You may not want to do this very often, or you may want to do it through your labour.

THE WAVE

You can do this visualization at any time during pregnancy or in labour itself.

Sit with your eyes closed and follow the movement of your breath as you breathe out and in. When you breathe out, lengthen your breath and allow it to drop into your abdomen so that as you breathe out, your abdominal muscles gently draw in. Don't force the movement.

The visualization

After a short while, imagine that each out breath is like a wave of water. Feel the wave beginning at the top of your head, and allow it to flow down through your whole body. Feel it flowing down the outside, from your head, over your shoulders and back, and down over your chest and ribs into your pelvis. Feel it flowing down through your pelvis and then over your buttocks and abdomen and into your legs. Feel it flowing down your legs and into your feet, then flowing out from the soles of your feet.

Now imagine that you can feel the wave flowing down the inside of your body, and focus on your main organs. Feel it flowing through your nose as your breathe out and in, and flowing through your lungs as they expand and empty. Feel it flowing through your heart as it beats, and through your intestines as cleansing water. Feel it flowing through your uterus and around your baby's body, and imagine your baby floating in the pool of water. Feel the wave flowing through your cervix.

In late pregnancy

You can begin to focus the power of the wave on opening up your cervix. With each out breath, feel the wave rushing through your cervix and opening it up.

In the last few weeks

Begin to focus on how you are going to use the wave during the contractions themselves.

Imagine each contraction coming into your body. As it grows in intensity it is like a wave rising in your body. It gets more and more powerful until it overwhelms your body, pounding it and beating it until you feel you can't breathe any more as you toss and turn in the torrent. Just as you feel you can't take any more, you feel the wave begin to die away. You breathe more slowly, and you begin to drift and float on the wave and feel yourself being washed towards the shore. You rest and relax, you float and you dream, your body lets go of the power of the wave. You float in the still water, at peace.

Then you begin to feel the wave rise again. You feel its power building inside you, surging in strength. It builds and builds. This time you imagine that you are in a boat, rising up with the wave. You reach the top and the boat is battered and thrown around by the building power and intensity of the wave. You rise and swirl, then gradually begin to come down the wave again to the peaceful water.

Now you feel the wave rise again, but this time you are on a surfboard. You have been waiting for the wave to come and you catch it excitedly, feeling its power and strength. You feel yourself being lifted up to the top of the wave, and find a point of balance and poise. Then you feel the sense of peace and power as you ride the wave to the peace of the shore.

When your contractions actually begin, as well as using the wave visualizations you might find it helpful to focus your attention on your cervix. As you feel the energy of a contraction beginning to build in your body, visualize your cervix gradually opening up. Imagine that you can see your cervix opening and thinning, as the contraction gets intense, and say the words "opening up, thinning out" as you breathe out during the contraction.

THE FLOWER

You also can imagine your cervix to be like a flower opening up, with its petals unfurling as the power of the contraction builds. With each contraction, picture the petals of the flower opening out.

TRANSITION BREATHING

Traditionally, transition breathing has been taught as a panting-type breathing, to slow labour down if your cervix is not yet fully dilated and therefore not ready for the second stage. I have not found this to be very helpful. This type of breathing doesn't really take away a premature urge to push — using the knee-chest position, which physically takes the pressure of

imagine that each out breath

is like a wave of water

the baby off the perineum, is far more effective. I also find that suddenly going into panting may tend to make mothers more anxious, and even prevent them from getting enough oxygen.

The most important thing during transition is to keep listening to your breathing and not give up the rhythm you have established. Transition may simply be a time when you need to rest and focus on your breathing in a calm way, but if transition is very intense, you will probably need to focus even more intently on it.

It is usually best not to change what you have been doing, if that has been working for you. However, if what you are doing isn't working, then you may want to try something different. If you are finding it hard to connect with the energy of moving towards the second stage, try the following visualization. It may help to calm you down.

TREE-ROOT VISUALIZATION

With each out breath, focus on relaxing down into your legs. Gradually begin to feel that your legs are like the roots of a tree, going down into the ground. Feel them burrowing through the earth and pushing further and further downwards. Feel the darkness and warmth and resistance of the earth. Feel the roots reaching right into the centre of the earth. Stay with this connection for a while.

SECOND STAGE BREATHING

It is still important to focus on the out breath during this stage, but now it has more power about it. As you breathe out there is a sense of strength behind the breath, which is helping you to focus your attention down to your pelvis, your cervix and perineum and help ease or push your baby out into the world.

You still need to stay relaxed as you breathe out. Often, a mother will feel that she is pushing or bearing down into her perineum, when in fact she is simply tensing her jaw, neck and shoulders and holding her breath in her throat. This makes for tiring and ineffective pushing. Instead, as you breathe in the second stage, you could allow your jaw to open and relax and use the open throat "aaah" sounds. As you do this, imagine that your breath is going down to your perineum and that you are using it to push your baby out. You can continue to focus on the tree-root visualization.

Images for the second stage

The kinds of images which may help in this stage include imagining your baby coming down your birth canal and moving out into the world, and visualizing your perineum opening and stretching. Some mothers find it helpful to physically hold on to a rope that is hanging from the ceiling. As they hold on with their hands, they imagine feeling the strength and power of the rope moving down into their body.

a growing shoot pushing up through the earth, like a baby pushing out through her mother's body

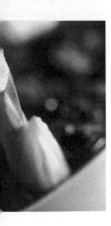

A GROWING PLANT

The image that best symbolizes the energy of the second stage is a shoot pushing up through the earth, like a baby pushing out through her mother's body.

As you breathe out more strongly, be aware of your baby's head coming down; allow it to emerge gradually out into the world. Think of your perineum as the earth surrounding a new shoot that is pushing its way through the ground in the springtime. Allow your perineum to stretch around the shoot, which is your baby's head. Be aware of your baby moving down the birth canal, and pushing through, like the shoot pushing through the soil. As you feel your perineum stretching and your baby's head coming out, breathe gently and don't push, and simply allow your baby to stretch your perineum. Let this happen gradually and don't rush.

THIRD STAGE BREATHING

Once your baby has been born, you need to keep your breathing focused until you have delivered the placenta. At this time you probably will be focusing more on your baby, but do remember to keep breathing deeply and to be ready for the contraction that will deliver the placenta. When this contraction comes, refocus and "breathe out" your placenta.

Placental visualization

Visualize how your placenta is attached to the wall of your uterus. Picture the blood vessels closing down and the placenta peeling away and gradually coming out, with minimal loss of blood.

FOURTH STAGE: BABY GREETING

Take the time after birth simply to be with your baby. Try to tune into how she is feeling now; imagine the big changes she is going through. Think about how you related to her when she was in your womb and how you are feeling about her now. She is the same person, even though that may seem hard to believe, and she will still respond to the things you said to her or the ways in which you related to her when she was in the womb. When my daughter was born, she was crying a little after the birth. My partner said her womb name "Little Fishy", and she stopped and stared wide-eyed at him.

Sit with your baby and touch her. Listen to her breathing and the rhythm of her breath. Notice how she is breathing compared with you. Focus on your own breathing rhythm and be aware of the differences between you.

Observe her movements. Try to imagine how she was curled up in the womb and now see how she is exploring the space around her.

Be aware of the sounds around you. The sounds and the voices of other people she hears are now are much louder than when she was in the womb but the reassuring sound of your heartbeat is not there. This is why a baby often loves being placed on her mother's chest. She can hear the sound of the heartbeat again, and that can reassure her. Place her on your chest and breathe together.

Talk to your baby, again remembering the way you talked to her while she was in the womb. Repeat her name to her. If music was important to you when she was in the womb, then play the same music to her now. She will love it. If there was a special place you went to in your mind when you were pregnant, talk to your baby about it. While you do this, you may want to keep her against your body, against your heart.

This is your personal time with your baby. Make the most of it; take time to enjoy her.

Physical preparation

Labour really is labour: it can be hard work. Bearing in mind that it is probably going to last at least seven hours, and that its end is the most physically demanding part, it is wise to have some physical strength to support you. That's not to say that you have to be super-fit to give birth; you just need to have looked after yourself physically during pregnancy and to have kept reasonably active.

In the last trimester, simply being pregnant and carrying all that extra weight around is working your body. How much extra exercise you should do, and what type, is going to be different for different mothers. What is most important is to listen to your body.

There will probably be days at the end of pregnancy when you feel tired – some more than others. On other days you may feel very energetic, but it is important not to use up all the energy in nest building or getting everything ready for the baby. You need to keep some in reserve to support you through the tired days. You also need to remember that life continues after birth. Your baby doesn't care as much about his nursery as having a relaxed mother.

You can incorporate practising the birth positions into a daily exercise routine, which will help keep your body in good physical condition for birth. They also help your baby to get into a good position. If you have been doing exercises during your pregnancy, some of these positions may be familiar to you. They are great to do

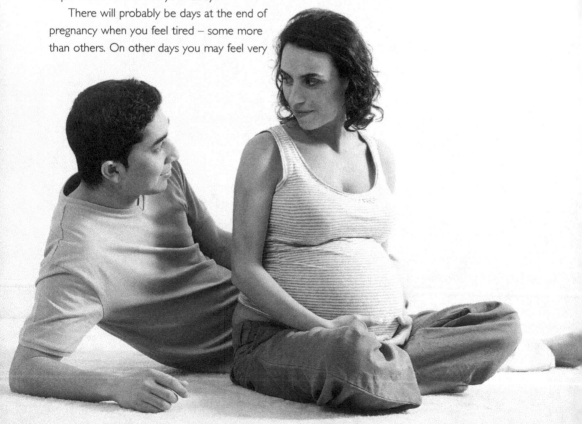

for the whole of the third trimester. If you find some of them hard, don't be discouraged; through practice, they become easier. Neither do you have to be able to do all of them, as long as you find one or two positions in which you feel comfortable. There is nothing to prove by being able to do them all!

Some of you might think that these positions are a little odd. When we see mothers giving birth in films they are usually lying on a bed. This is one of the worst positions in which to support the natural process of labour although it may become necessary if medical intervention is needed. By laying down, your sacrum (the flat bone at the bottom of the spine) cannot move and a lot of pressure is placed on it, so labour tends to be more painful. Secondly, you are working against gravity. That makes it harder for your baby to come down onto your perineum in first-stage labour, and during the second-stage bearing-down, you are working against gravity, in effect pushing your baby uphill. Thirdly, by leaning back you encourage your baby to be in the posterior position, which may result in a more difficult delivery.

Some mothers worry that being in these positions might be undignified. But which is more dignified – to be on all fours giving birth, or lying on your back in stirrups while someone pulls your baby out with forceps? Your baby has got to come out one way or another, and it is up to you to decide whether you want to work with your body as much as you can or rely on others.

Your birth partner

It is important for your birth partner to practice these positions. Labour can be hard work not only for the mother but for the partner as well. If a partner is going to give good physical support then he also needs to be in fairly good physical condition, or at least know his limitations. There is no point your partner becoming injured during the labour by putting his back or knees out while trying to support you in an awkward position. Apart from not being so great for your partner, he won't then be able to continue to support you in labour, nor help you postnatally nor enjoy being with your new baby.

Your partner needs to be able to support you with the minimum strain and effort on his part. This means learning to be in tune with his body. Your partner also needs to be able to

Physical awareness combined with relaxation is key for the partner as well as for the mother

COMMON FACTORS

All the suggested birth positions involve movement of the pelvis, the use of gravity, and leaning forward. These positions also will help in the last trimester of pregnancy, by easing lower back tension and helping your baby to engage and settle in the preferred anterior position.

Pelvic movement

These positions allow your sacrum and your pelvis to move as they need to move during labour to allow your baby to go down the birth canal and be born. If you put pressure on your sacrum, as you would if you were lying on your back, this limits its movement. Suggested positions include lying on your side, leaning forward on your hands and knees, or squatting. You can sit, but only if you sit in such a way that you are not directly on your sacrum – for example, sitting the wrong way round on a chair, or on a ball.

Use of gravity

Helpful birth positions make use of gravity, which helps your baby to move down in your pelvis, and, in turn, helps to stimulate contractions. This means that generally you are in an upright position or on all fours, rather than lying down.

Forward leaning

The emphasis in the positions is on leaning forward, which helps your baby stay in a favourable birth position (head down and spine away from your spine) as well as taking pressure off your lower back, which will tend to ease the pain.

do this so that he can give effective massage. If your partner is uncomfortable in any way, then this is going to transmit into his touch, which then won't be so beneficial for you and may even feel unpleasant.

Using a birthing stool

Giving birth is amazing and may even be spiritual, but it is also closely linked to basic bodily functions, and it is important not to deny that aspect. The nearest experience you may have had to giving birth is going to the toilet, and some mothers do in fact give birth on the toilet.

A birthing stool is really a version of a toilet seat. This is quite a helpful idea to work with, because if you are going to the toilet, you don't want to sit on a flat surface (you need space beneath you) and it is hard to eliminate if you are lying on your back.

When you practise your birth positions, you could use the toilet seat in place of a birthing stool, but it's much better to use your partner's legs – they will be a lot more comfortable than a hard seat! You can sit on your birth partner's lap with your thighs on his (see page 33); that way you keep your sacrum and perineum open.

PREPARING TO PRACTISE THE POSITIONS

The positions are essentially the same for the first and second stages of labour, and to some extent the third stage, if you want a natural delivery of your placenta. The main difference is a switch of emphasis.

During the first stage, the emphasis is on relaxation and on opening up the pelvis. In the second stage, the emphasis is on bearing down with a little more effort and focus. In both stages it is important to use the space in between contractions to rest and gather your energy, both physical and mental. For each position, I

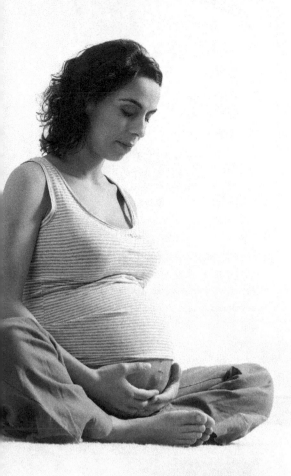

For the third stage, you would tend to use the same emphasis as for the second stage, but this stage is not as intense. The placenta often comes away without much effort and you may deliver it while lying down.

The fourth stage is about bonding with your baby, so you simply need to choose whichever position you are most comfortable in. By then, you will probably feel like lying down maybe on your back and propped up with cushions so that you can feed and touch your baby.

You should do the following exercises with your partner, if possible, but you also can do them on your own. During all the exercises, use the basic deep-breathing technique. When you are in labour, you will be working with both breathing and position so you need to practise this in advance. Remembering to breathe deeply also gives your body the maximum physical benefit from the exercise.

If you want to modify an exercise slightly, feel free to play around with it, but if either of you feel any discomfort during an exercise, please don't continue with it.

give a more active Yang version, which you will probably use more during a contraction, and a resting Yin version, which you will tend to use between contractions.

First stage labour

The emphasis is on relaxation and opening up the pelvis – moving hips

Active versions: use during contractions

Resting versions: use between contractions

Movement from Yin water, to Yang water: the waves increasing in intensity, opening up, going with the flow, relaxation, surrender.

Second stage labour

The emphasis is more on bearing down

Active versions: use during contractions

Resting versions: use between contractions

Yang wood: the shoot pushing through the earth, downward movement, perineum opening up.

Third stage labour

The emphasis is similar to the second stage, but not as intense

Active versions: use during contractions

Resting versions: use between contractions

Fire: stay focused, connection and bonding.

Bonding with your baby

Choose whichever position suits you best; you may want to lie down

Fire to metal: creation of two more distinct identities: connection and communication.

STANDING EXERCISES/ FIRST STAGE PRACTICE

The basic standing exercises are suitable for most mothers in late pregnancy.

Dancing

This relaxing position tends to be fine for most mothers.

ACTIVE VERSION

Stand facing your partner, with your feet about hip width apart. Hold hands and be aware of each other's breathing. Breathe out and in together (1).

After a while, begin to rock and sway together. You can rock from side to side (2 & 3), or do some circling movements with your hips (4). You can even put some slow music on and dance along to it. Play around with different movements, focusing on the rhythm.

Take notice!

Don't try any of the more demanding positions, especially the standing squat, if you have (or suspect you have) any of the following:
• symphysis pubis problems
• knee or ankle problems
• vaginal bleeding or a low-lying placenta
• your baby is breech.
The simple rocking movements will be probably be fine, but be aware of how you feel. It is important for both of you to be comfortable and not to strain, so don't do any movements if you are unsure about them. If your partner has knee or ankle problems, he also should avoid the more strenuous exercises.

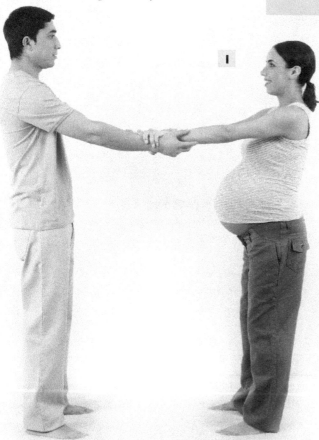

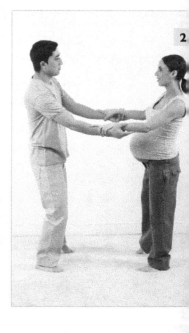

Some people say that Arabic dance originally developed as a birth dance. In Arabic dance, hip and pelvic circling movements are important, and images of snakes were often used to portray the flow and rhythm of the dance. You could imagine that you and your partner are amorous snakes twisting and turning to a snake-charmer's music.

You can then practise circling around and taking each other's weight, as you lean back (5). However, you should not do this if you have symphysis pubis problems.

RESTING VERSION

Imagine you have been dancing and now feel really tired. Just lean into each other's arms and rest (6). Practise the slow deep breathing together, and see how much you can relax while standing.

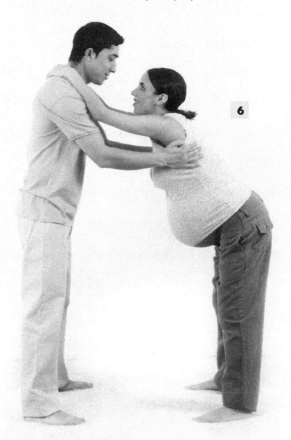

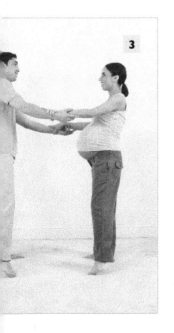

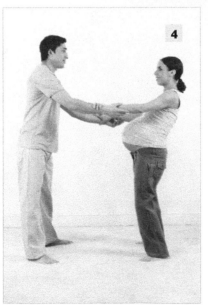

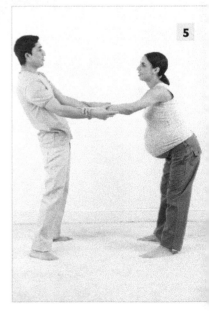

Standing squat

Physically, this is a more challenging exercise than dancing. To do it, you squat down slightly, not into a full squat but just taking your weight down to the point at which your thighs are roughly parallel to the ground.

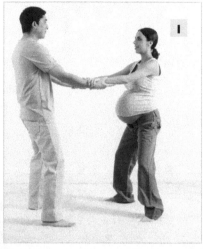

ACTIVE VERSION

Stand completely straight with your feet as far apart as feels comfortable, and your arms fully extended and holding your partner's wrists (1). Breathe out slowly while sinking down together and taking each other's weight (2). Once you are in the squatting position, you can try rocking a little from side to side (3 & 4). Please make sure that the centres of your feet are carrying your weight and that your knees are in line with them. If you let your knees fall inwards, you risk putting too much strain on your ankles.

RESTING VERSION

When you are in the squatting position, hug your partner and lean forward onto him. Both of you can rest in this position, practise your slow deep breathing, and really let go and relax. You also could get your partner to lean against the wall or sit on a chair while you sit on his thighs and rest.

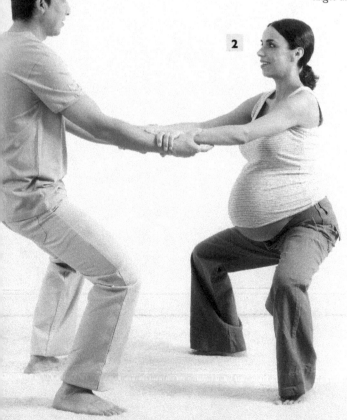

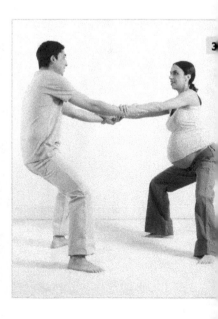

STANDING EXERCISES/
SECOND STAGE PRACTICE

The exercises are essentially the same as for the first stage, but you should get your partner to take a little more of your weight, as though you are giving birth. Try to bear down as you imagine you would in the second stage of labour. He may need to lean against a wall to support his back, or sit on the edge of a table or chair or on a birthing ball.

This is also where your partner can be like a birthing stool and you can sit down on his thighs. You can either face your partner or have your back to him but it's vital that he is completely relaxed and doesn't feel any strain. You may need to play around a little with these different positions, to find which of them works best for you.

Resting standing squat
Your partner needs to adopt a position that is comfortable.

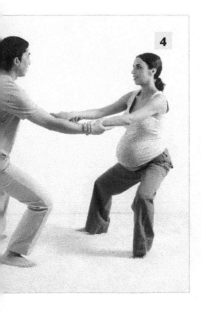

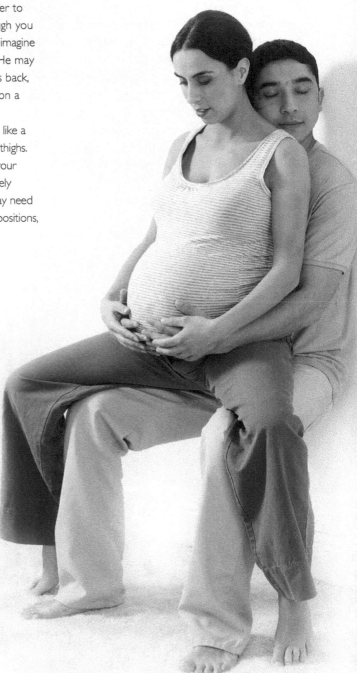

ALL-FOURS EXERCISES

These are great exercises to practise and usually you don't have to worry too much about precautions. However, if one person is much larger than the other, he or she should always be the supporting partner and remain underneath. Do be careful, too, if either of you has a wrist problem such as carpal tunnel syndrome (soreness, stiffness or tingling in the wrist); pressure on your wrists may aggravate it.

If this exercise proves to be uncomfortable for your wrists, then you can adapt it by leaning over a ball or chair instead of crouching on the floor on all fours.

When you do these exercises, make sure that your lower back is flat and not hollowed. If it is hollowed, you will put too much strain on both your lower spine and your abdominal muscles. You also need to check that your knees are comfortable and that you have enough padding under them.

It is a great position for helping your baby get into the anterior position, and it will help a breech baby to turn. It also strengthens your abdominal muscles, allows your pelvis to move, and gives your lower back some temporary relief from carrying the weight of your baby.

First stage

ACTIVE VERSION

Make sure that the surface on which you are going to work is not too hard (not a bare floor) but not too soft either. If necessary, use a thick rug or a yoga mat, but not a physio mat because these are usually too cushioned and will harm your wrists. One of you (it doesn't matter which, but you could start with whoever is bigger) gets into the all-fours position while the other one leans over his or her back.

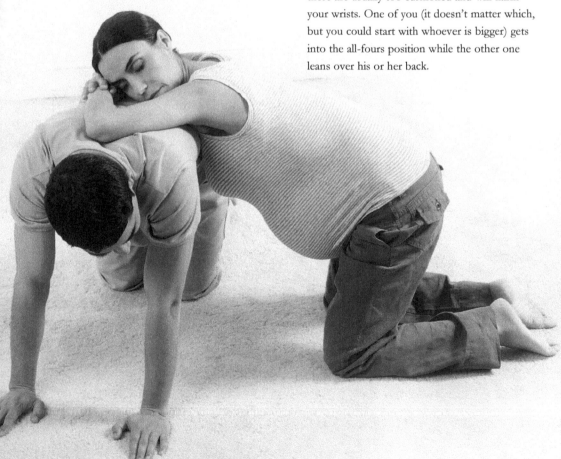

When you are the one doing the leaning, make sure that you spread your weight evenly over your partner's whole back, not onto the middle. To do this, rest one forearm over the upper back and the other over the lower back, especially over the sacrum.

Imagine that your partner is like a soft ball and begin to move together using your hips. You can rock backwards and forwards and do more circling- type movements. The person on top can lift one leg up and do some more circles into that hip (NB don't lift your leg if there are pubic bone issues). After a while you can change hips and use the other one. You also can lift yourself up and take more of your weight on your forearms. Then you can swap who is underneath and who is on top – provided there is not a large weight difference. It can be a good way for the partner to practise relaxing while the mother is moving around.

After a while both of you can try resting. The person underneath needs to relax as much as he or she can while the person on top totally relaxes and flops. Often the person on top is worried that his or her weight will be too much, but if it's spread and the weight difference is not enormous, it feels comfortable for the person underneath. Indeed, it is also a good introduction to the massage work, because a lot of the techniques for labour involve the partner simply leaning their bodyweight in a relaxed way, onto the mother. If the partner is really tired but the mother still wants some physical contact, he can use this position to rest over her. The partner gets to rest while the mother gets some good contact.

Second stage

This is essentially the same as for the first stage, but the person on top needs to lift up a little and imagine that he or she is bearing down with some force, instead of flopping over the one underneath. You can practise both a resting and an active version of this.

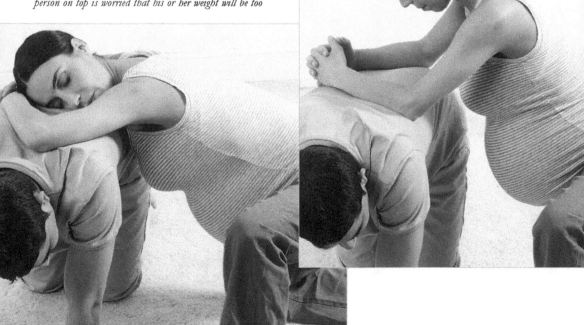

Knees-to-chest position

This is another, more restful variation on the basic all-fours position. To get into this position, start on all fours then come down onto your forearms and have your bottom higher than your head. Make sure that you don't hollow your lower back. If you have a cough or heartburn, this position won't be so comfortable, but usually it's very restful.

USING IT IN PREGNANCY AND LABOUR

In pregnancy, this can be a good position if you have symphysis pubis pain or a low-lying placenta because it takes the pressure off your perineum and pubic bone. It may also help a breech baby to move their head down or a posterior baby to move their spine away from the mother's spine.

During labour, you can use this position in either the first or second stage when you want to slow labour down.

You might wonder why you would ever want or need to slow labour down. The reason is that some mothers – sometimes even first-time mothers – have very quick labours and the whole thing is over in a couple of hours or even less. Usually, this is actually quite traumatic for the mother. She doesn't have time to get into a proper rhythm, and everything is over before she has really gotten into it.

This also can be a useful position in which to take a break if labour is very intense. It will take the edge off painful contractions, but bear in mind that it does this by slowing labour down. Therefore, if your labour is long, adopt this position for just a limited time if you want to give yourself a break.

Another time it can be useful is when you feel that you want to bear down during transition, before you are fully dilated. If you bear down on a cervix that is not fully dilated, then you can cause it to swell so it can't open any more. Your midwife will warn you if you try to bear down too soon. You might even have a sense yourself that bearing down isn't helpful.

If you use the knee-to-chest position, you will take the pressure off your cervix and this will stop you wanting to bear down. It is usually more effective than the panting breathing that is sometimes taught for this situation. However, if you still feel you need to bear down even when in this position, it is probably because your cervix has now dilated fully.

This is also a good position for a mother to use in second stage if she is bearing down but nothing seems to be happening. Sometimes this happens because the baby is stuck in the wrong position. Rather than continuing to bear down and forcing the baby into even more of a stuck position, the mother can adopt this position to take the weight off her perineum. This can give the baby a bit more space to move back slightly, adjust his position and then come down again in the right way.

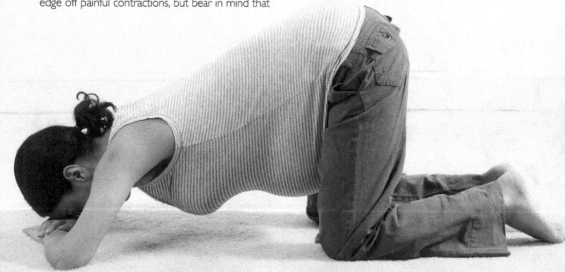

SQUATTING EXERCISES/
FIRST STAGE PRACTICE

These are the exercises that have the most precautions attached to them, and the ones that are hardest for us in modern societies where we tend to do a lot of sitting in chairs and not much squatting. Squatting is one of the ways people sat before there were chairs, and how they went to the toilet. We can see how natural a position it is when we go to countries where it is still very much used, and when we see how our own toddlers squat with ease.

Squatting strengthens your pelvic floor, helps your baby to engage and may ease sciatica and lower back problems. It also may help relieve constipation. It is a great position in which to givie birth because it opens up the bones of the pelvis, giving the widest diameter for your baby to come down through, and uses gravity in the strongest way.

If you are not comfortable with the squat then don't force it, but you may find that with practice it becomes a very comfortable position for you to use.

To do the exercises with your partner, you must both feel confident about going into the squat. You should each try going down into the squat on your own and seeing how far you go and how comfortable you are. To do this, have your knees about hip width apart and sink down into the squat from standing. Alternatively, you can start off on all fours and then rock back into the squat. You may find you can't quite make it, so try a little rocking from side to side.

Sometimes, shifting your weight around will help you to go into the position. See if your heels go down onto the floor easily or not. If not, you can put some books or cushions under your heels to make it more comfortable. You need to make sure that your weight is over the centre of your feet and you are not letting your ankles collapse in. To help with this, you can place your palms together in front of you and ease your elbows against your knees, to keep the pressure off the insides of your ankles.

If you can't do the squat together, you can try going down into the squat by holding on to the back of a chair or a door handle and sinking down. When you try the exercise together, you should be giving each other a similar kind of support to the chair or handle.

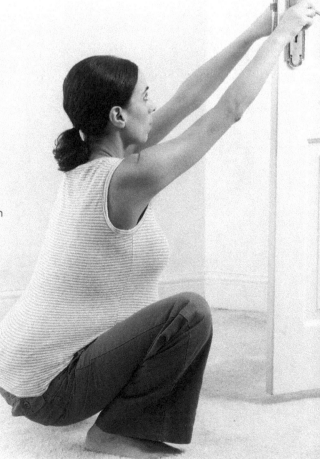

Partner squat

ACTIVE VERSION

Stand facing your partner, making sure that your arms are fully extended and your back is straight, as in the standing squat (see page 32). Have your legs about hip-width apart. As you both breathe out, keep your arms extended and sink down into the full squat position. Don't worry about overbalancing. If you both do this properly, you will each get support from the other.

Once you are both down in the squat, you can try rocking a little together. Stay in this supported squat position for as long as you both feel comfortable, but leave yourselves enough energy to come up together, reversing what you did to go down.

Take notice!
Don't try any of the squatting exercises if you have (or suspect you have) any of the following:
- hemorrhoids or varicose veins: the pressure will block circulation, making it feel uncomfortable
- your baby is breech: squatting will push your baby's bottom deeper down into your pelvis, making him more breech and less likely to turn. If your baby is in a good position however, the squat will help his head to engage
- symphysis pubis problems; the exercises will aggravate the pain
- a low-lying placenta or any placental bleeding; the exercises may put undue pressure on the placenta
- any discomfort or pain in your knees when you try to squat.

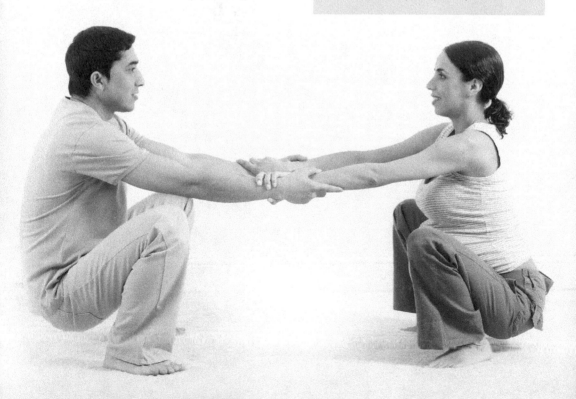

*With practice and when you get used to it, you may well
find that the squat itself is a very comfortable position and
one in which you can rest. If it is not, try to find a way
of taking some of the pressure off being in the squat so
that you are resting more. This could be taking the weight
forward and into your arms, leaning on the floor or leaning
back slightly or resting your back against a wall. You could
also put cushions under your heels. Your partner could sit
on a chair or ball and you can rest against him. You could
either have your back to him and be more upright or face
into him and lean more forwards. Experiment to find what
feels right for you.*

SECOND STAGE

This is essentially the same position as
recommended for first stage practice, but try to
imagine that you are bearing down.

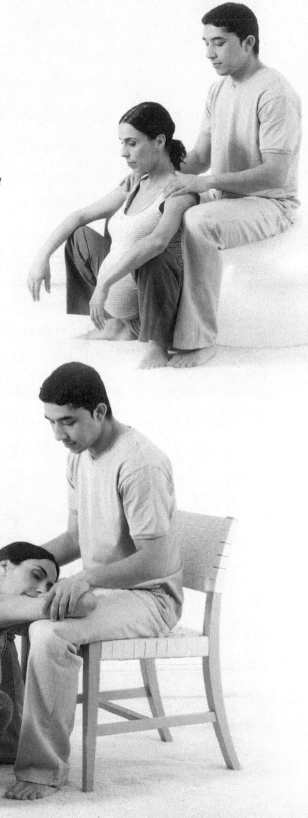

SITTING EXERCISES

Although you really can't give birth sitting, many mothers find that sitting at some point during the first stage or transition can be a good resting position. However, you should try not to sit in a normal way on a chair, because it will put pressure on your sacrum and encourage you to lean back, so here are some alternatives that you can use during that stage.

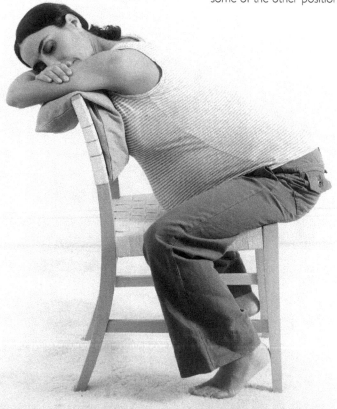

Sitting backwards on a chair

Sit the wrong way round on an armless chair so you are facing its back. You will need to open your legs around the chair, so don't do this if you have symphysis pubis problems. Make sure that your coccyx is off the end of the chair so that no pressure is being applied to it. If you like, you can put a pillow or cushion over the back of the chair so that you have something comfortable to lean over.

Take notice!

If you have pelvic pain then the sitting backwards on a chair and the sitting rocking on a mat exercise may be too much, because they involve opening up your legs. You can still try the sitting on a birthing ball version.

Sitting in a rocking chair

Rocking chairs are quite comfortable during the second stage, because as you rock back and forth, you are not putting a constant pressure on your sacrum. You put pressure on it only when you rock back, not when you rock forward. Many mothers find that using a rocking chair is very relaxing, especially for a labour that has a long latent stage. As labour gets more intense, though, they usually need to get up and use some of the other positions.

Sitting rocking on a mat

This is quite a fun exercise to practise with your partner, but don't do it if you have symphysis pubis problems. It is a good position for early labour, but as labour progresses, there is usually too much pressure in the perineum for it to be comfortable.

Sit on the floor, on your mat, with the soles of your feet together and allow your knees to come down towards the ground. You can do it on your own, or sit opposite your partner and do it together. Try to sit upright with a nice straight spine, and hold on to your feet or ankles. Now begin to rock gently from side to side. Don't rock too quickly or you might feel a little unsettled, and don't rock too far over or you might lose your balance. Start with a nice gentle rocking movement and focus on finding your rhythm.

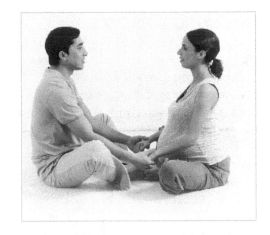

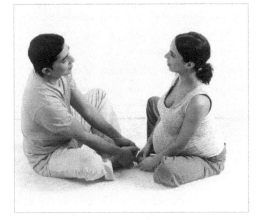

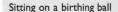

Sitting on a birthing ball

Using a ball is good because you can sit on it without putting pressure on your sacrum, you have to sit upright, and you can rock around on it. You can also move easily from sitting on the ball to leaning over it on all fours.

SIDE-LYING EXERCISES

Side-lying is the most restful and least active of the positions. It doesn't use gravity or promote movement in the same way as the other positions, but is a great relaxation position to use at any point in labour when you feel tired. It is much better than lying on your back during labour, which apart from slowing things down, is usually extremely uncomfortable.

Side-lying even can be used as a position in which to give birth to your baby if none of the others seem to be working. Midwives often like mothers being in this position as it is easy for them to see what is happening with the baby.

If you have been practising the other, more active, positions, this is a good one with which to end your practice as you can both lie down together.

First stage

Lie down on your mat on one side, whichever side feels more comfortable. Place cushions where you feel you may need them, such as under one leg, or between your knees, or under your abdomen, chest, or neck. This is where the big breastfeeding cushions can be great to hug. Now your partner can snuggle in next to you. He can lie behind you, with his abdomen against your back, hugging you and maybe even placing his hands on your abdomen. You could rest in this position doing the baby breath hug together.

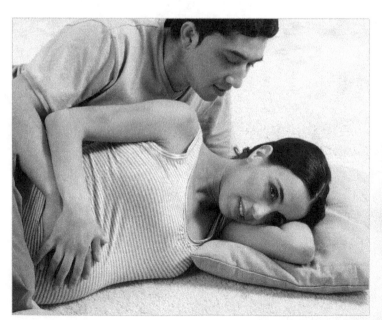

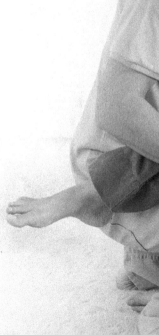

Second stage

You may need to prop yourself up on one arm a little. Your partner gets up and holds your foot so that you can push against him, imagining you are bearing down.

PELVIC FLOOR EXERCISES

You may have been practising these already during your pregnancy, but during the last few weeks you can begin to emphasize the letting-go aspect of them. This will be helpful during both the first and second stages.

Going down to the basement

Breathe in and out slowly, and at the start of an out breath contract your pelvic floor around your vagina. As you continue to breathe out, gradually draw the muscles up deep inside as though they are going up in a lift. Draw them up to the first and second floors, then keep going to the third and fourth if you can. As you breathe in again, hold the muscles drawn up. Then when you breathe out, let them go back to the third, second, first, and ground floors and then even lower, down to the basement. Feel the letting go. How much can you let go?

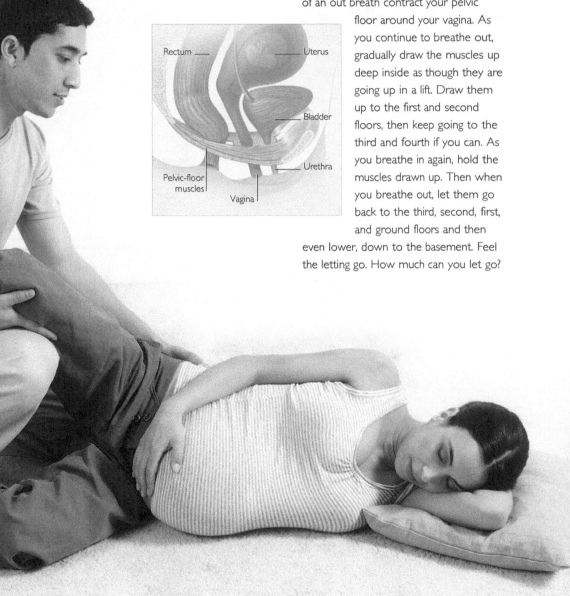

Rectum — — Uterus

— Bladder

— Urethra

Pelvic-floor muscles

Vagina

Using positions in labour

Practise and play with the basic positions until you and your partner both know them well. You need to feel that you can move together, almost as if you are dancing, because birth is like an improvised dance. While you can practise certain movements, you don't know how they will link together on the day. You may find that while pregnant you prefer certain movements, but when you are in labour you prefer others.

You need to make sure that both you and your partner are comfortable in the positions. Obviously, in labour it is your partner that has to follow your lead, but he must make sure that he is as comfortable as he can be in his supporting position. You may find that you want him to give you lots of support, or very little, or there may be times when you just want to be on your own in one of the positions.

During labour, you may find you use lots of different positions or maybe there will be just one that you enjoy using. It is good to practise all the different positions though, and try linking them together. How do you move from the squat to all fours? How do you get from standing to side lying? Try to maintain a smooth, dance-like flow as you move from one position to another.

You also can practise doing the "going down to the basement" for your pelvic floor exercise in each of the positions. Notice in which one you can let go the most.

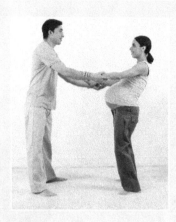

STANDING

Like many mothers, you might like to stand during early labour. You just can walk around, then stop and sway your hips as you need to. You also could try leaning over the side of the bed or against a wall. Many mothers find that they then need to try other positions, such as on all fours, but some do give birth standing up.

As labour progresses, you might find you need more support from your partner. He will need to lean against a wall, or sit on a chair, to be able to support more of your weight as you bear down.

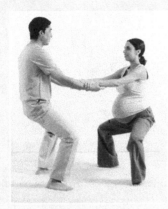

STANDING SQUAT

Some mothers use the standing squat in the first stage of labour, and it is also a great position for the second stage if you are not feeling that in touch with bearing down. This position helps the baby come down the birth canal and gives you a sense of what you may need to do for bearing down – even if used for only a minute or two. Some mothers, may even give birth in this position, so it is important to make sure that someone is there to catch the baby.

You might want support from your partner, but he does need to make sure that he is supported as well, by standing against a wall to support his back or by sitting on the edge of the bed. You can use his legs like a birthing stool and sit on them, making sure you are taking your weight on your thighs and not compressing your sacrum.

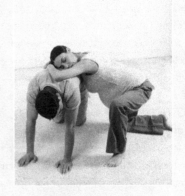

ALL FOURS

The all-fours position is probably the one that most mothers feel most comfortable with for a lot of the time during labour. It is very versatile and not tiring to be in, and it can easily become a resting or an active position. Your partner doesn't usually have to give that much support in this position, which makes it easy for him to give you some massage if you want it.

You can use the all-fours position during the first stage or second stage, and use the knee-to-chest version of it to slow labour down, if necessary.

MAKING USE OF HOSPITAL EQUIPMENT

Whether you intend to give birth at home or in hospital, it's a good idea to visit the hospital once you know the kind of positions you like. See what kind of furniture they have that you can lean on, and what you might need to bring should you have to go there to give birth. Some hospitals have birthing balls and yoga mats, some don't. Even if they do, they might be in another room when you need them, and it is often comforting to have some of your own things around you in a hospital setting.

USING THESE POSITIONS IN WATER

If you are thinking of using water in labour, either for pain relief in the first stage or indeed to give birth in, I suggest that you first practise the breathing and the different positions in a swimming pool. Then, when you finally get your own birthing pool, if you are going to give birth at home, practise them again there.

You can use most of the positions in a pool, and the squatting positions are a lot easier there because you are supported by the water. Lying on your back in water can actually be both relaxing and beneficial at any time during late pregnancy. You are not compressing your sacrum and so you are not going to feel pain, and the baby will tend not to move into the posterior position while he has the space.

In water, as on dry land, you need to feel comfortable in the different positions and in moving from one position to another, so take the positions and play. You could even try going under water and seeing how you feel with that – some mothers go under the water and hold their breath between contractions. I find this is a good example of doing whatever works for you.

Of course, you can't do the side-lying or knee-to-chest positions in water, but to slow labour down, you can lean back and float a little.

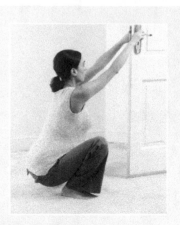

SQUATTING

This is the strongest position in that it both uses gravity and allows the pelvis to open up the most. However, it is the position in which you are likely to need the most support. Some mothers find they like to use the side-to-side rocking movements in early labour and during the first stage, but most save it until later on unless they are really comfortable in the position. You can hold on to a door handle or the side of the bed to get support, or get your partner to help you. He could be sitting on a chair or maybe using the ball, and you could use him like a birthing stool.

Whatever you feel
like doing is fine;
there is no right way,
only the way
that works for you.

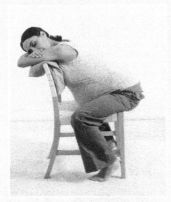

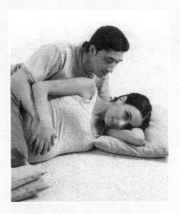

SITTING

This is usually more a position for early first stage labour. You can use it as a resting position and then get up and move into other positions as you need to, but when you are using it, always make sure that you're not putting pressure on your sacrum. A good way to avoid this problem is to sit on a birthing ball, or the wrong way round on a chair.

SIDE-LYING

This is great for when you feel tired, as it is not as active as the standing or squatting positions. You can use it, pretty much as you practised it, at any stage of labour when you feel you need more of a rest.

SYMPHYSIS PUBIS PROBLEMS

Pelvic pain: many women suffer from some pain or discomfort in the pelvis in pregnancy. The cause is the weight of the baby plus the hormonal changes which lead to a greater softness in the tissue. This means that the joints of the pelvis have more pressure put on them and can move more. We must remember that greater movement of the pelvis is important to give space to the baby and to support birth and is a natural change. Why then do some women experience pain? It can be for many reasons: hypermobile pelvis before pregnancy, weak abdominal and pelvic floor muscles, poor posture, previous injury. It is important for each woman to work out which movements and positions help ease pain and which aggravate it as they are different depending on the cause. Good posture is always helpful (tucking the pelvis under and engaging the abdominal and pelvic floor muscles) and movements which reduce weight in the pelvis (e.g. knee to chest or all fours). Movements which move the joints in the pelvis may or may not be helpful. The main message is listen to your body and work out what helps and what doesn't.

Massage and shiatsu

Having some form of massage during labour can bring you many benefits. It is a way to involve your partner, so that he can give you real support and connect with both you and your baby. It may provide effective pain relief and comfort, and give another focus to your breathing so that you are able to relax and work with your contractions. You also can include your baby in the massage, which can help both of you to enjoy the beautiful experience of birth.

Many mothers find they enjoy being massaged so much that they don't want their partners to stop, even to have a drink, but others only want massage from time to time. Some may not even want it at all, but that is often because they are being massaged in the wrong way or the wrong place. However, once mothers find what they need, most love being massaged. But partners must respect a mother's wishes if she doesn't want to be touched. Sometimes a mother just wants to go into her own private space.

Shiatsu

People often think of massage as lots of stroking. While labouring mothers usually like some stroking and rubbing, there is so much going on internally that many find this irritating, especially during contractions. What pregnant women tend to prefer are the holding and pressure techniques that are more a part of shiatsu.

Shiatsu is a form of massage that involves acupuncture points and meridians as well as muscles and blood flow. Applying pressure to certain shiatsu points can be a powerful way of providing support to a mother in labour (see box, opposite page). The meridians each relate to the five elements: note the colours on the chart. Refer back to chart on p 21.

Practising makes perfect

It is important that you and your partner practise the massage techniques before you go into labour, and learn how to do them in the different birth positions. That way, you can familiarize yourself with them and have some idea of the ones you may want to use during the birth.

It also can be fun for you to practise on your partner, who is not going to get any massage when the big day comes! When you practise massage on your birth partner, it can help him to understand what the massage can feel like and is a lovely way for you to connect with each other. It also could reveal whether your partner feels comfortable with massaging you. If the answer is no, you might want to consider getting someone else to be with you during labour to provide the massage aspect of support. You could contact local shiatsu or massage practitioners about this, and find one who has specifically trained in labour work.

Make sure you have a few sessions with your chosen practitioner before the birth, to check that you feel comfortable with each other. You should also ensure that your partner feels comfortable with having someone else there during the birth, and agree in advance how you are all going to work together.

Guidelines for birth partners

When you give someone a massage, particularly an expectant mother, it is always much more enjoyable and effective if you follow some simple rules. Below are the basic guidelines that all birth partners need.

Shiatsu

A non-invasive technique, this is a type of massage originally developed in Japan based on Chinese medicine integrating with their traditional massage anma. It aims to boost the body's self-curative abilities and can relieve pain, reduce tension, promote relaxation, rebalance the body and maintain good health. The most well-known form of acupressure, shiatsu involves using the hands, fingers and thumbs to stimulate key pressure points on the surface of the recipient's skin. It is traditionally done through clothes, but can be done directly on the skin. Traditional Japanese midwives used it in their work. Suzanne was fortunate enough to work with a Japanese midwife in London whose grandmother was a midwife in Japan. Modern shiatsu was introduced to the west in the 70s and has evolved with an integration of our anatomical awareness of the body. Shiatsu continues to evolve as our understanding of the body evolves, but it is fundamentally rooted in the eastern energy view of the body.

MERIDIANS

These lines are pathways carrying energy (known as qi or ki) from the principal organs around the body. There are 12 main ones, which relate to the different organs and their elements. The points along them can be worked to balance the energy from the area of the body through which they pass. There are also two central channels – Governing Vessel and Conception Vessel. These regulate Yin and Yang energy and overall flows. They have a particular connection with the womb and regulate fertility, pregnancy and childbirth.

PRESSURE POINTS

Key points, also known as tsubos. are located on the meridians through which energy flows. Pressing or holding a point can stimulate or calm the energy inside an entire meridian. Some have particular uses for labour.

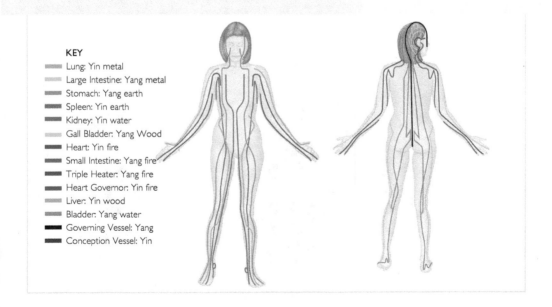

KEY
- Lung: Yin metal
- Large Intestine: Yang metal
- Stomach: Yang earth
- Spleen: Yin earth
- Kidney: Yin water
- Gall Bladder: Yang Wood
- Heart: Yin fire
- Small Intestine: Yang fire
- Triple Heater: Yang fire
- Heart Governor: Yin fire
- Liver: Yin wood
- Bladder: Yang water
- Governing Vessel: Yang
- Conception Vessel: Yin

CORRECT BODY POSITION

When you are giving a massage, make sure that you are in a comfortable position so that you don't get tired or tense. If your body is tense while you work, this tension will transmit itself to the mother, undoing much of what you are trying to achieve.

Achieving a comfortable body position and fluid, tension-free movements are other good reasons for practising the birth positions and breathing exercises. To give a massage properly, for example, you need to move from your hips a lot, so all the hip-circling movements you are practising are great as preparation for that. You also may be spending a lot of time standing or kneeling while you are massaging during labour, so prepare for this by practising the standing and all-fours exercises.

Another essential is to make sure that your shoulders are relaxed. This, in turn, will help you to keep your elbows, wrists and hands relaxed and, especially if you are applying pressure through the thumbs, to keep your thumb joints straight or supported. If your thumbs are bent and you use a lot of pressure, you risk straining their joints.

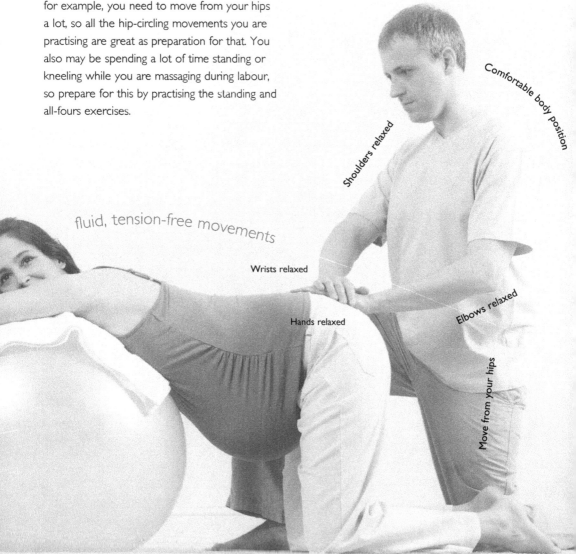

fluid, tension-free movements

Shoulders relaxed

Comfortable body position

Wrists relaxed

Hands relaxed

Elbows relaxed

Move from your hips

WORK WITH THE BREATH

Both partners need to incorporate working with the breath into the massage sessions. The mother is going to experience deeper relaxation if she can breathe deeply. For you, breathing deeply will help you to be more relaxed in your work, and your relaxation will, in turn, transmit to the mother. Deep breathing also encourages a connection between the two of you.

USING YOUR HANDS

Although it may not be possible with some strokes and routines, always try to keep both hands in contact with the mother's body with holding and pressure techniques. If one hand is still, that will give the mother a more secure and comforting feeling (Yin hand).

Stroking

When you stroke, you can stroke slowly or quickly and firmly or lightly, and the direction of the strokes you use will depend a lot on what you are trying to achieve with them. If, for example, you are working to support blood circulation in the body, then downward strokes away from heart are more calming and strokes towards the heart are more stimulating.

If you are working to support blood circulation in the limbs, especially the legs, you should use the firmer strokes going towards the heart, so as not to put any undue pressure on the vein walls. If the mother has varicose veins, only ever touch lightly, simply moving the skin but not compressing the vein.

If your focus is to work along the energy lines or meridians, then generally you should work down the back of the body and down the backs of the legs to the feet. When you work on the front of the body, work up the insides of the legs but, in pregnancy, down the front of the body to the abdomen.

Pressure techniques: shiatsu work

When you use the static holds you can be very versatile in the amount of pressure you use. You can work so deeply that you feel you can't lean in any more, or your touch can be as light as a feather. The pressure is determined by what the mother wants, and it can vary as labour progresses. Generally, mothers want more pressure as their contractions get stronger, but some mothers may want a lighter touch. And some may not want to be touched at all.

Most of the time, you should apply the pressure at 90° angle to the body. This is so that it is a nice, deep, penetrating pressure that doesn't pull at the skin and muscle. Sometimes, though, the shiatsu points are under bones, so the angle will have to be slightly different so that the pressure can reach the point.

Holding the points

You can maintain your pressure on the shiatsu points for as long as it feels right. This might be for only a couple of minutes, but during labour it could be much longer – even hours.

It is important to remember that the way in which you touch areas and specific points is as important as locating the correct position of a point. If you are working specific shiatsu points you should stimulate them when the mother breathes out, so it is helpful for both of you to breathe together.

Stimulating the points often works best during contractions, when you should increase the amount of pressure as the intensity of contractions increases. In between stimulating the points, which is usually in the space between contractions, do some stroking movements, either light or vigorous, or apply a lighter general pressure. This can be relaxing for both you and the mother.

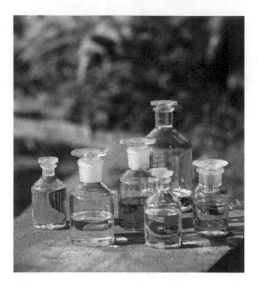

Take notice!
Aromatherapy oils are powerful medicinal oils that can overstimulate the body. If you want to use aromatherapy oils for your massages, first ask a qualified aromatherapist specializing in birth work to recommend oils that will be safe for you to use.

USING OIL

You can use all the techniques that follow either through the mother's clothes or directly on her skin using oil. Some of the techniques are shown with oil and some without, but you can do them whichever way you both prefer. Some mothers like to spend labour with most of their clothes on, others don't.

In pregnancy it is advisable to use oils that are as close to nature as possible, as the body absorbs a percentage of everything put on to the skin. Always use a vegetable oil such as olive or sunflower. Neal's Yard Remedies have developed a range of natural products with a base of nourishing cold pressed oils such as almond, sunflower and borage; these also have subtle natural fragrances. Alternatively, use a beeswax-based product such as the Tui waxes from New Zealand; with a wax, there is no risk of spillage.

KNOWING WHEN TO STOP

While you should both enjoy using all of these techniques, not all mothers will like the same things and on some days one or both of you might feel like different kinds of work than on others. The basic guideline is that if something doesn't feel quite right, then stop. Maybe it is not the right technique for you, or maybe you aren't doing it correctly. You could try a few variations, but if it still doesn't feel right, please stop and seek advice from a qualified massage therapist.

MASTERING THE TECHNIQUES

Practise all the different techniques as much as you can before labour. You will probably find that the mother likes some techniques more than others, which may be an indicator of what she is going to prefer during labour. However, you can never predict exactly what kind of massage she is going to want then, so it is best to practise everything with which she feels comfortable.

Make sure that you practise the massage techniques along with the birth positions. Practise them more with the positions you both prefer, but, unless you really can't do or don't like a position, try to practise all of them.

With each technique I indicate when and why it will be most effective, but. in fact. you can use any of them at any point during labour – just respond to what the mother wants; she knows best, provided she is in touch with her body and her baby. If she is feeling stressed or disconnected, then try different techniques and pressures until you find what helps her feel more in touch and relaxed again. Many of these techniques also may be of benefit by helping the baby move into a good position during the birth.

USE DURING LABOUR

When you are massaging the mother during labour, the most important thing for you to do is to respond to what she says, such as "harder", "gentler" or "not there". She will let you know what is right, and it is hard to do something wrong because she won't let you. Don't feel criticized if you keep being told to do something differently; the fact that she is asking you to do it at all means that it is helping. If she says nothing, then assume that what you are doing is correct. She won't necessarily respond in the way she might do when you are practising, saying things like "that's nice", or "that's relaxing". And don't expect her to thank you for what you are doing! The best response in labour is for her to be able to continue and to focus. In between contractions she may want to talk to you about what you have been doing, but she may instead just need to rest.

Usually, it is during the first stage that mothers want most to be massaged, and typically they want more and stronger massage as the contractions get stronger. The area most mothers want to be worked during contractions is the lower back, especially the sacrum. Next in popularity is the abdomen. However, some mothers prefer the arms and hands or legs and feet, and others the neck. Some want lots of different things, while others just want one point held for the whole of labour.

In the second stage, the mother may want you to continue with what you have been doing so far, but most want to be touched less. Some, especially if the first stage has gone well, find that they need to focus inwards to deliver the baby and do not want to be touched at all. However, in the second stage the neck and shoulders, and maybe the jaw, tend to get really tense, so working on these areas can be helpful. And if the baby is getting a little stuck, then it can be useful to work on some of the labour focus points to try and help him move.

As with everything in labour, what mothers want varies hugely. As the partner, don't feel that you have to try to use everything you have learned and practised. You may use it all, you may use none of it. Probably you will use some of it. If it works, do it. Don't see any of the practice as wasted, because if the mother and baby enjoyed it during pregnancy, it was well worth doing.

Even if you don't get to use much of what you have learned, you will have prepared yourself to feel confident during the mother's labour, and gained skills that you can continue to use afterwards. Mothers and babies continue to benefit from massage after birth, and continuing with some of what you have done, and using it as a basis for adding some new massage skills, can form an important part of a great system of family support and communication.

it is hard to do something wrong
   because the mother won't let you

Massaging the back

One of the main areas in which mothers feel tension, pain or discomfort during labour is the back, especially the bottom of the back – the sacrum. This is the triangular bone at the base of the spine. It is attached via the sacro-iliac joint to the hip bones, which in turn attach to the pubic bones at the front. The tops of the hip bones are called the iliac crests, and the bottoms are the ischial tuberosities (the sit bones). These are the main bones of the pelvis, and will move or open out slightly during labour to allow a baby to pass freely down the birth canal to be born.

GETTING IN TOUCH WITH THE PELVIS

The following routine is for both partners to understand how a woman's pelvic bones move, and how their movement can be affected by different birthing positions. Before trying it for the first time, both partners should explore their sacrum and pelvis using hands and fingers.

Place your hands over your sacrum and feel your coccyx, the knobbly bit at the bottom, then move your hands up and feel the flat of the sacrum or triangular bone. See if you can feel how wide it is and if you can detect any of the holes. Compare the feel of your sacrum with that of your partner's.

Now feel around to your hips and to your pubic bone at the front. Then feel underneath your hips to your sit bones at the bottom.

Now the mother is ready to discover how her pelvic bones move when she is in different birthing positions.

To begin, the mother stands in front of her partner who places his hands on her buttocks. Then the partner gently pulls his hands back, so that she can feel the lower part of her pelvis start to open.

Next, she sits down and feels the distance between her pubic bone and her coccyx, then leans forward into the all-fours position and feels the distance between the two bones again.

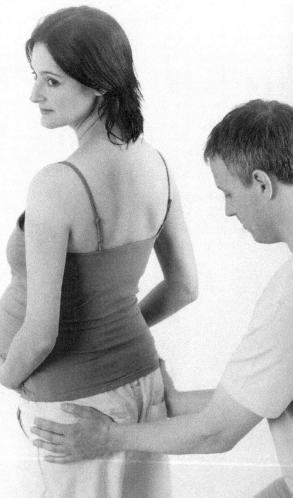

Finally, if she is able to go into the squat, she moves into that position and feels the distance betweeen the bones again.

Each time she moves, she should feel that the distance gets a little bigger. It is not a big amount, but even a few millimetres in labour makes a huge difference. This is why the different birthing positions are so important.

IN LABOUR

Sometimes in labour, the baby may get a little stuck as she moves down the pelvis. If the mother uses the different positions she has practised, this tends to help minimize the chances of the baby becoming stuck, but it is good to have a couple of techniques that a partner can use to really open out the pelvic diameter. I am indebted to my shiatsu colleague, Anna Moonen from New Zealand, for showing me these, which were developed by the Pink Kit team in that country.

With the mother lying on her side, the partner can exert some pressure into the centre of her buttocks and open them out (1). You also can try this when she is in other positions, such as standing or on all fours. Feel how this pressure opens out her hips.

If the midwife is supportive, or you have another birth partner to help you, at the same time as one of you is opening out the hips, the other can apply some pressure to the sacrum, gently pressing down to the feet (2). When you do this, the mother can really feel how her pelvis opens. This movement can help her to feel less scared when she experiences the natural opening of her pelvis at the end of the first stage and during the second stage of labour.

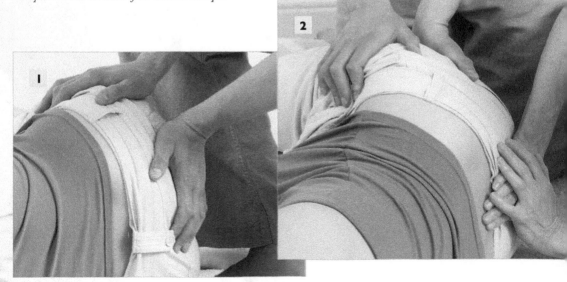

SHIATSU FOR THE SACRUM

Because mothers often feel pain in the lower back and sacrum when the baby is pressing against it, massaging this area may be helpful during all stages of labour, Both firm, slow stroking and applying pressure can be very effective at relieving pain. A partner can apply pressure in a general way, or work on the four pairs of points in the bony indentations of the sacrum. Applying pressure during a contraction directly relaxes the area as well as the whole pelvis, and can provide pain relief while allowing labour to progress.

Sometimes, mothers like the pressure to be continued between contractions, although usually not as intensely. Lighter general pressure, or gentle stroking over the lower back or maybe down the legs, between contractions, can help aid relaxation and the conserving or renewing of energy, allowing the mother to get ready for the next contraction.

Having the mother on all fours is a great position in which to practise, but during labour, you can try it in any position in which you can access the back. These are good techniques for a woman to practise on her partner, so try to do them sometimes that way round.

Sacral pressure

It is possible to apply very strong pressure on the sacrum and this is usually what mothers want, but don't overdo it. Use only the amount of pressure your partner needs.

You can use this technique during the second and third trimesters of pregnancy, so

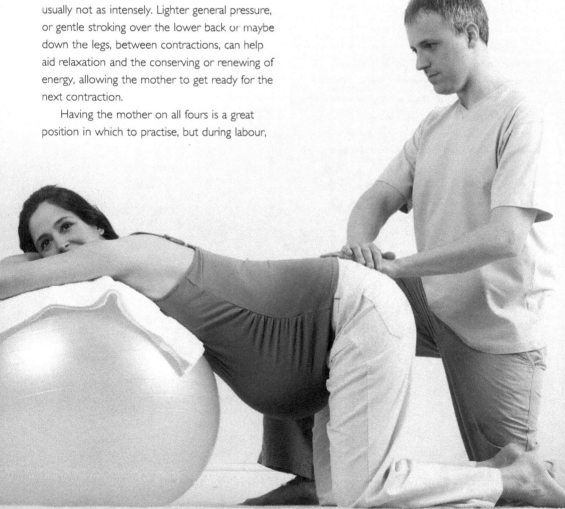

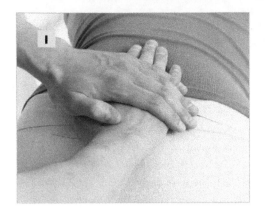

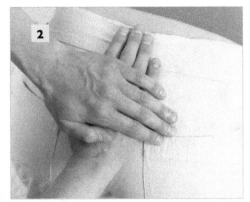

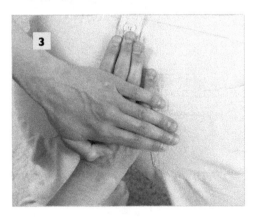

long as you are sensitive to how much pressure the mother wants. Usually, as her baby gets heavier and more weight is placed on her lower back, she will want increasingly stronger work. However, some mothers may want really deep work from the middle of the second trimester onwards, while some may want light pressure even in labour.

Start with the mother leaning over a ball or a chair. If she is leaning over a ball, it is probably a good idea to place a cushion in front of it to stop it from rolling too much. You could also use the cushion in labour if the mother doesn't want to move too much. Placing a towel or blanket over the ball can make it a bit more comfortable. If the mother is leaning over a chair, put a cushion over the back of it to make it more comfortable.

You also need to find a comfortable position in which you can reach the sacrum. Depending on your height, you could either stand up or kneel by the mother. The most important thing is that you can lean your weight forward into your hips, so that any increase in pressure is applied by leaning more body weight onto your arms, rather than pushing down from your shoulders. Your shoulders must be completely relaxed as you work, because giving pressure from your shoulders usually feels quite uncomfortable for the mother and can be very tiring for you. Once you find a suitable position, you can use it for all the sacral work.

Start by placing one hand on top of the other in a criss-cross pattern, with the fingers of the lower hand facing up the mother's spine. Relax your hands and allow them to mould to the shape of her body. Begin applying pressure at the level of her hips, and maintain it for a few breaths to find how much is comfortable for her. Make sure that the pressure you apply is at an angle of 90° to her body (1).

Now slide your hands down an inch or so and apply the pressure again (2). Repeat this until you are at the bottom of the sacrum, which is the coccyx (3). When you have applied pressure there, go back to the original position and start the process all over again. Repeat this a few times, gradually building up to the maximum pressure that is comfortable for the mother as you do so.

During labour, work on whichever area on the sacrum feels most comfortable for the mother. This usually varies as labour progresses. In early labour, for example, she might like the pressure to be high up and not very strong, then as labour progresses, she might prefer you to work further down and more deeply.

The pressure that the mother wants in labour is likely to be a lot stronger than whatever you were using during pregnancy, and she will usually want even greater pressure as her contractions increase in intensity. Some mothers like fairly constant pressure both during and between contractions, but others like the pressure during contractions and some other holds or stroking techniques in between them.

Sacral opening and gathering

A mother can often experience discomfort because of a build-up of tension in the sides of her sacrum and in her buttocks. Working directly on these areas will release the tension and ease the discomfort.

You can apply pressure to each side of the mother's sacrum in two different ways. One is by sacral opening, in which you ease the pelvic bones away from the sides of the sacrum. The other is by sacral gathering, where you ease the pelvic bones towards the sacrum. Usually one way feels better than the other, especially if the

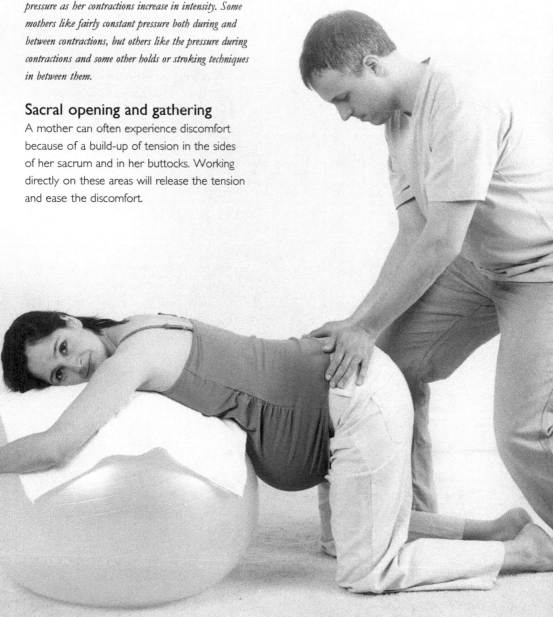

mother has any problems with her sacrum. Just use the one that she prefers. You also can put this kind of pressure into each buttock. Either put one hand on each buttock and apply pressure with both hands, or put one hand on top of the other on one side at a time.

Using sacral opening or gathering may be a good way to relieve backaches, especially those caused by the sacro-iliac joint. It also may help the mother to focus her attention to either her back or her front.

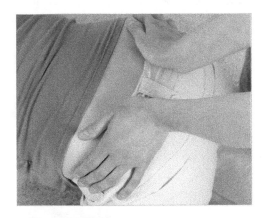

SACRAL OPENING

This technique gives the mother a feeling of support in her pelvis, and can feel great if she has symphysis pubis problems. It also helps her to focus her attention to her front.

THE PRACTICE

Place your hands on the mother's lower back with your fingers pointing out, and align the heel of each palm along each edge of her sacrum. Lean forward and down, and at the same time drop your elbows out so that you open up the sides of her sacrum. This small movement helps to bring her pubic bones slightly together at the front.

SACRAL GATHERING

This works in the opposite way to sacral opening, and helps the mother to focus on her back. Do this cautiously if the mother is suffering from symphysis pubis disorder because it may aggravate the condition.

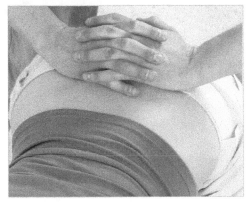

THE PRACTICE

Place your hands so that your fingers are pointing to the centre and the heels of your palms are still along the edges of her sacrum. Your hands may overlap. As she breathes out, lean down and slightly squeeze your hands together. This brings energy into the sacrum and opens up the area around the symphysis pubis.

IN LABOUR

These techniques can give good relief from sacral discomfort. Mothers often like having pressure here for quite a lot of the labour, both during and between contractions.

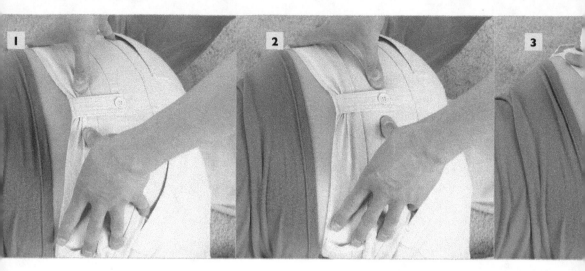

Sacral groove work

Although the general pressure of sacral opening and gathering can be very effective during labour, sometimes it is not enough. When that happens, it can be helpful to apply strong pressure into the grooves of the sacrum, with the mother in the all-fours position.

This work is usually great in later pregnancy, but don't do it in the first trimester (while the baby is forming) because it is quite strong, releasing work and doesn't usually feel appropriate. There isn't a lot of pressure on the sacrum at that stage of pregnancy, so it is not particularly needed. In labour, however, this pressure may be very intense and sacral groove work is often very helpful during contractions.

THE PRACTICE

The sacral groove pressure points are two sets of four holes in the sacrum. There is one set on each side of the sacrum's midline, usually about a thumb's width out from it, although that varies from person to person depending on the size of his or her bones. On some people, the points are easy to find, but on others less so. You usually can locate them by feeling from the hip bone,

following its curve down until you reach the top points. Alternatively, locate the tail bone (coccyx) and feel up for the lowest set of points.

To work the points, begin at either the top (1) or the bottom (2) and place your thumbs in a pair of points. Start gently massaging around the dip with small circling movements. This allows your thumbs to settle in the centre of the point. Then lean in with your body weight (by leaning from your hips) to apply static pressure. Make sure that your shoulders are relaxed and your thumbs are straight.

To increase the pressure in the points, you can work them one at a time. Place one thumb on top of the other on the point and lean in deeply (3). Make sure your fingers support your hand by making contact with the mother's body. You can also use your knuckles in these points, either one at a time (4) or in pairs (5).

Whichever method you use, always work all four pairs of points. You may well find that some points are easier to feel than others, some may feel tender to touch, and others you press into quite deeply. Work first with the points that feel more comfortable. You may find the mother wants you to stay there, or that she finds one side

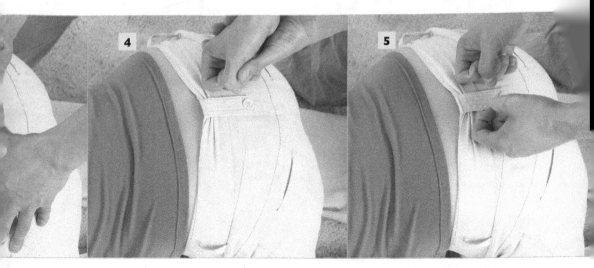

is more comfortable than the other, or maybe that she prefers certain pairs of points. Work on them for as long as the mother wants you to.

You can use the same technique with the mother lying on her side but you will need to kneel down to do this. Face her body and work the grooves on the side that is uppermost. You also can do this when the mother is standing, but the pressure you will be able to exert will probably be a little less.

Once you are comfortable doing this work with the mother in a static position, practise with her rocking and moving. She can use her body as she moves to push into you.

After working on the sacrum, it is a good idea to do some hand-over-hand stroking over her buttocks and down her legs, and finish by holding her feet. This will allow the energy that has been released to flow and be integrated by the rest of her body. This feels very relaxing for the mother and in labour it feels almost as if you are drawing the pain or discomfort of the contractions down and out into the ground.

You can do the stroking either through her clothes, or directly on her skin with oil. Try both ways and see which she prefers. Begin working with light strokes, then try heavier ones, then work slowly and then quickly. In this way you can discover which combination of pressure and speed she likes. While you are stroking, make sure that your wrists are completely relaxed.

IN LABOUR

This deep sacral work is probably the technique most favoured by mothers in labour. The strong pressure helps release tension from the sacrum and also gives a focus to the breathing. Many mothers find that this is all they want through the whole labour, and they like it both during and in between contractions. Usually they like the more intense pressure as the contractions get stronger, and enjoy a release of the pressure in between contractions.

Other mothers like strong pressure during the contractions and either very little or no pressure in between them.

STROKING DOWN THE WHOLE BACK

The gentlest form of back work is simply to stroke lightly down the whole of the mother's back, from her shoulders to her legs. This is a hand-over-hand stroking and it can be done as firmly or quickly as the mother wants. It can be done through the clothes on directly on the skin if you use some oil.

The effect is almost as though the strokes are drawing away the pain

THE PRACTICE

Start at her shoulders, then stroke down over her spine and buttocks and down onto the tops of her thighs. This can feel calming to her if the strokes are slow, and stimulating if they are quick.

IN LABOUR

During labour, mothers usually prefer to have their backs stroked in between contractions rather than during them. The effect is almost as though the strokes are drawing away the pain.

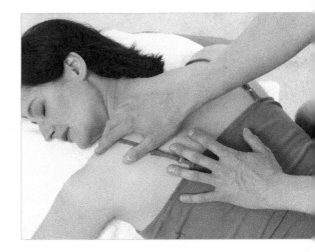

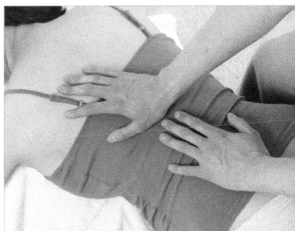

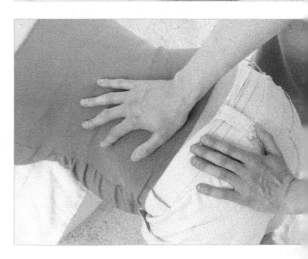

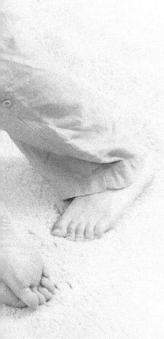

Massaging the abdomen

In many traditional cultures, a mother's abdomen is massaged a lot both in pregnancy and in labour. Often the work is vigorous with techniques to move the baby into a good position before labour and during labour itself to help move the baby if he or she gets stuck.

Modern mothers, however, would find many of these techniques uncomfortable and some are not particularly safe either. Women in traditional cultures typically engage in work that is physically active, such as digging fields, carrying water or washing clothes in rivers. Their abdomens tend to be well toned and strong. Many modern mothers, on the other hand, spend a lot of time sitting down, do their work at a desk, and drive cars; their abdomens,

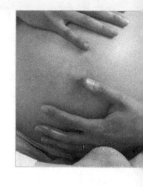

therefore, often are not particularly strong. Massage, however, can help support the abdominal muscles and bring more of a connection to this area including a greater awareness of a baby.

In our culture, we are often overly protective of our abdomens. When women are not pregnant, they don't often want their abdomens to be massaged but somehow, when a woman is pregnant, even strangers will feel it is all right to come up to her and pat her tummy. While this does not feel appropriate, there is something positive about the pregnant abdomen that makes people want to touch it, and it is a lovely way for family and friends to bond with a new baby.

Pregnant women often instinctively rub their abdomens, especially later on as their babies get bigger, although some mothers and partners are unsure as to how much they can rub. Sometimes parents feel afraid of touching the abdomen for fear of harming the baby so it is worth thinking about how deep a pressure the midwife uses when she is feeling for the position of the baby in the last trimester. Her pressure can be uncomfortable, but shows how well protected the baby is by the amniotic fluid, the uterus and the abdominal wall. It would be a bit of a design fault if the baby was so vulnerable you couldn't touch her.

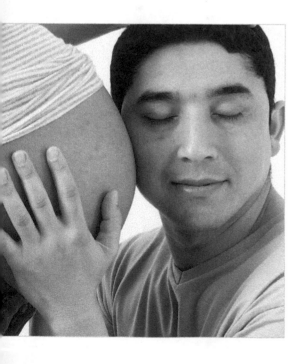

In pregnancy

You and your partner, and even other children, can rub your abdomen to connect with your baby. You can rub through your clothes or rub in lots of oil on a bare abdomen. Oil, especially one rich in vitamin E such as wheat-germ, can be great for nourishing the skin.

You even can use strokes to encourage your baby to move if he or she isn't in such a good position. These needn't be very vigorous – just gentle encouragement rather than forcing her to move. It is good to combine touch with breathing and with talking to your baby, either in your head or out loud. This type of work is often very effective in helping your baby to change into a better position for birth.

In labour

Mothers will either love or hate touch of the abdomen during labour. Massage can feel very reassuring; the feeling of hands on a mother's abdomen may help her to focus on her breathing and enable her to breathe deeper and to concentrate more on her baby. This helps bring a more positive focus to labour as it takes the mother away from the pain of the contractions. A mother even may use the techniques during labour to help her baby move.

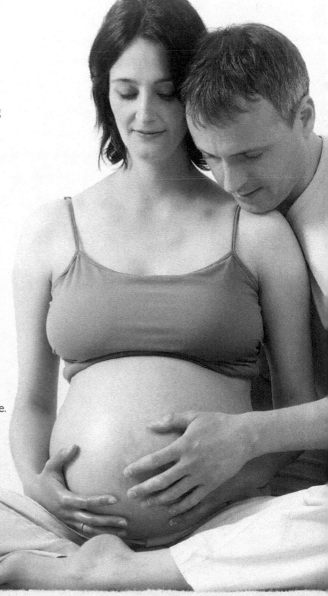

GENERAL ABDOMINAL PRESSURE

This gentle but effective massage technique often is pleasant and comforting for the mother, and a great way for her and her partner to connect with the baby. It is also one of the few techniques that a mother can do by all by herself, if she wishes.

THE PRACTICE

Although the mother being in the all-fours position is a good one in which to practise this technique because that is often the most helpful during labour, the partner can do this with the mother in a variety of different positions. She could be lying on her left or right side – depending on her preference – or she could be sitting or even standing. For the partner, the main thing is that you are in a position where you are comfortable and you can have your body close to her's. One of the easiest positions is with the mother sitting, and you sitting behind her.

The massage can be done either through her clothes, or you can rub some oil directly onto her bare abdomen before massaging it. If you are rubbing in oil, begin by warming it in your hands and then gradually smoothing it over her abdomen with sweeping clockwise strokes. It is important to work in a clockwise direction,

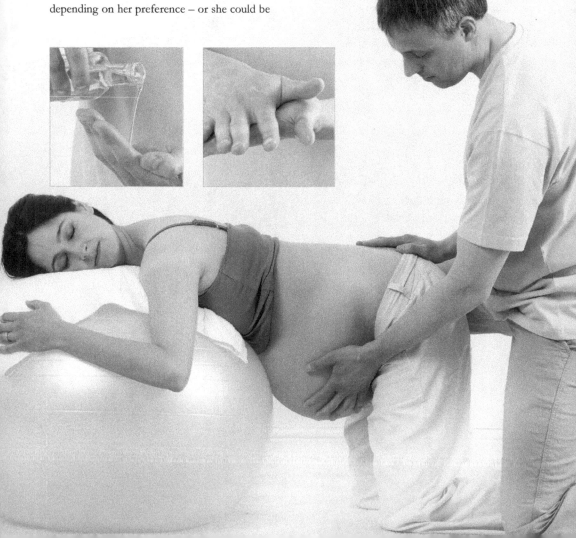

because then you will be following the movement of the intestines.

Now place one hand on her abdomen and the other on her lower back. How high or low on her back you place this hand depends on what is most comfortable for the mother. Having it somewhere on her lower back tends to allow her to feel less invaded and more supported, and to experience a connection that is deep inside her body from front to back.

Just allow your hands to mould to the shape of her body and rest there for a while. Be aware of the baby in the womb. Feel the connection between your hands and the movement of the mother's breathing as it draws your hands gently together while she breathes out and gently pushes them away again when she breathes in. After a while, begin to apply gentle pressure by drawing your hands together as she breathes out. When she breathes in and you feel your hands being pushed away, release the pressure but maintain the contact.

Keep the hand you placed on the mother's back still throughout the exercise, because it gives her lovely support. Move your other hand to work different places on her abdomen. To move that hand to a new position, slide it through one or two hours in a clockwise direction around the abdomen. When it reaches a new place that you want to work, repeat the pressure as before, but remember that the amount of pressure you can exert will vary from place to place.

You may also find that some places draw you in and you want to work on them for longer – it is fine to spend extra time on these. Other places may feel firmer and perhaps seem to push you away, so that you only want to stay for a few out breaths.

The way the baby responds to the massage will often change as you apply the pressure to different areas. He might perhaps follow your hands around, or even kick you.

IN LABOUR

Abdominal work can be especially good in early labour. It may help the mother connect with her breathing and to breathe deeper, which can help her to focus on her baby rather than her pain. It may help to calm the baby especially if he has been used to the mother's and partner's touch. A mother even can use it to help her baby move.

Of course, there may be times in labour when a mother doesn't want any contact with her abdomen, and for some mothers this could be throughout labour. However, many mothers do appreciate their partners holding their abdomen – sometimes even for the whole of labour.

Self massage

You can use abdominal massage as a great way to communicate to your baby.

See if you can become aware of different parts of your baby's body. You probably won't be able to tell if you are touching a foot or a hand, but you will be able to feel the little limbs pushing into you. You might not be able to tell the bottom from the head, but you will be able to feel a hard lump, and you will probably be able to work out what is the spine and back – this will be a larger, flatter area. You may find that as you touch different places, your baby will move around.

You can use self massage to help your baby get into a good position for birth (see page 116). Ask your midwife to tell you your baby's position and to teach you how to identify the position yourself. If your baby's head is away from your pelvis and is in the breech position, see if you can feel how to ease his head down gently towards your pelvis. You shouldn't use strong pressure while you do this – it's more about just using your intuition. If your baby's spine is facing your back, for example, you can gently stroke from back to front while talking to him, in order to encourage your baby to bring his spine around. If you make a good connection with your baby, you will sense how you need to stroke and hold.

Even if your partner is going to massage you, you may feel happier starting the session with some self massage to help you connect with your baby. You can do the baby breath hug (see page 17) with your hands on your abdomen, and with each out breath allow your hands to draw in as deeply as you feel appropriate.

The kidney womb hold

This technique is similar to general abdominal pressure, but this time the hand that you place on the mother's back must be over one or the other of her kidneys.

THE PRACTICE

Each kidney is mostly tucked under the ribs, so cup the hand that is on the mother's back over her lower ribs on one side of her spine. Visualize energy from the kidney beneath your hand moving through into her lower abdomen. Move the hand that is on her abdomen and apply pressure with it as before, then move the hand on her back to cover her other kidney and repeat the process. Can you feel a connection between your two hands? Maybe you have a sensation of warmth, maybe it simply feels pleasant and comfortable for your and the woman, and maybe an image of some kind arises within you.

IN LABOUR

This technique gives a more specific focus to the abdominal work by centring on the kidney, which in Chinese medicine relates to sending powerful replenishing energies to the womb. At any stage of labour, it can be especially helpful during times when the mother is completely exhausted, or when her contractions seem to be ineffective. It may also be a useful technique for calming a distressed baby.

Supporting the pelvic girdle

You can try this technique in many different positions, but a good one is with the mother on all fours, perhaps leaning over a ball or a beanbag. You can do this with her fully clothed, or use oil and work directly on her bare skin.

THE PRACTICE

Stand or kneel, depending on your height, with your body behind the mother and your abdomen, which is going to give support, close against her back. Place your hands over the centre of her abdomen either above or below her navel, depending on which is the more comfortable for her. Being supported quite low down – just above her pubic bone, where her abdomen starts to round out and the muscles and ligaments are quite stretched – will often feel good to her.

As the mother breathes out, gently draw your hands towards her back. Then, with a firm stroking movement but without pulling on the muscles, move your hands from her front to her back. Pass them around her hips, ending up at about the level of her second or third lumbar vertebrae and drawing the energy from her pubis to her back. Focus your mind on the inside of her body as well as the outside, so that a deep connection is made, then focus on the baby. Rest your hands on her sacrum to finish the first part of the massage. Next, starting from the sacrum, repeat all those actions in the reverse order, sliding your hands from back to front. Some mothers are clear that they prefer the

movement in one way only, while others enjoy both directions. For mothers with symphysis pubis disorder, however, it is usually best to draw the energy from the back to the pubis, as there is often a lack of energy here. As this is not a strong opening technique like sacral opening (see page 59), it also can be used the other way, if there is too much energy in the front. You can repeat these movements as many times as you and your baby enjoy them, exploring moving slowly and a little more quickly.

IN LABOUR

The mother may find this a very calming and reassuring hold, one that can help her focus on her breathing and on her connection with her baby. If she feels more discomfort in her abdomen than in her sacrum, you can focus on drawing the pain from the abdomen round to the back. If the pain is more severe in her back, draw it round to her abdomen.

Some mothers may like this hold all through labour, but others may find that as labour progresses, they don't want to be held around the abdomen so much. Some appreciate this hold more during a contraction, while others prefer to be held in between contractions.

THE KIDNEY WOMB HOLD (BELOW)
SUPPORTING THE PELVIC GIRDLE (RIGHT)

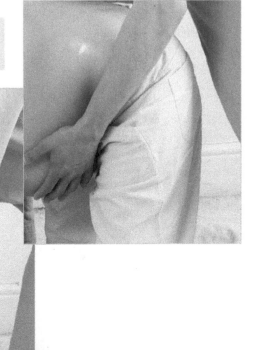

Shiatsu and massage for the head

These are important areas to work on because they are common sites of tension. In labour, mothers often clench their jaws and tighten their shoulders. This can give rise not only to generalized tightness in the neck and shoulders, but also to specific symptoms such as headaches, nasal congestion and emotional tension. In shiatsu, the pressure points in the side of the neck, the tops of the shoulders and around the shoulder blades relate to the gall bladder meridian, which is associated with wood energy. Wood energy is related to strong physical downward movement and the delivery of the baby so neck and shoulder work is often used to support second stage labour.

The neck is closely related to the sacrum, being at the other end of the spine. Sometimes, if it feels too intense to work the sacrum, then the mother may enjoy having her neck worked. It is possible to relieve back tension by working the neck. It is even possible to help shift the baby, if he is in an unfavourable position. The points on the sacrum are bladder points and so are some of the points on the neck, so working on the neck helps keep water energy flowing as well as wood energy. Water energy dominates the first stage of labour while wood is the driving energy in the second stage. In the five element cycle (see p 21) water nourishes wood.

Usually, a mother will enjoy this work, but if she has suffered any neck injury then even very light pressure and holding may feel uncomfortable. If this is the case, don't do any work on her neck.

It is also a good idea for the mother to use these techniques on her partner, because many people, even those who are not pregnant, have neck and shoulder tension.

SHIATSU POINTS

Below you will find how to access the various points, situations in which to use them and ways to them work effectively.

I BLADDER 10 (BL10)

There are two points – one each side of the neck; working them may help relieve tension in the back of the neck, headaches and sinus congestion.

To locate the points, place your thumbs each side of the neck vertebrae, about 1½ thumb widths from the centre. Slide up to the base of the skull. There you will find a hollow at each side of the neck, about half an inch above the hairline and in the slight depression about an inch to each side of the spinal groove.

Work these points one at a time, using your right hand to work the left-hand point and vice versa. Hold your thumb in one side, with the fingers of that hand resting comfortably on the mother's head. Put your other hand on her forehead and use it to guide the head into the thumb. Because the points lie under the back of the head, then instead of exerting pressure at a 90° angle, you need to angle your thumb so as to hook under the bone parallel to the spine. Do this slowly, building up pressure gradually to the amount of pressure the mother feels comfortable with. When you have finished working that point, change hands and work the point on the other side.

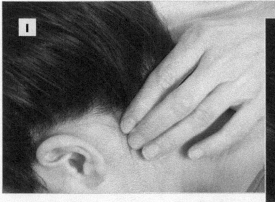

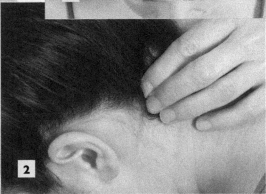

2 GALL BLADDER 20 (GB20)

Working these points helps to release tension in the head, especially tension relating to headaches in the side of the head. It helps to ease tightness in wood energy, so it is especially helpful in second stage labour.

These points lie at the back of the head, an inch above the hairline in the depression between the muscles on each side of the head. Locate Bladder 10 (see opposite page), then slide up and slightly out until you come to a protrusion of the skull. The points lie just below this protrusion. These points are just above and to the outside of the two Bladder 10 points.

Work these points in the same way as Bladder 10, except that you need to angle the pressure in at 45° (diagonally) while hooking under the bone.

3 GOVERNING VESSEL 20 (GV20)

This point, right at the top of the head, is the highest point of the body. Known as the "point of a hundred meetings", it is on the central meridian, which regulates yang or outward-moving energy and hormonal energy. It is a very good hormone balancing and calming point and good for regulating blood pressure. Working it at any time the mother wants you to will help to keep labour flowing.

To find it, place your thumbs on the tips of her ears and extend your middle fingers towards each other – it is one thumb-width in front of where your middle fingers meet. This is usually just in front of the crown of the head.

To work this point, place one thumb on top of the other over the point and cup the head with your hands and fingers. Your thumbs are going to be working and your hands will be acting as support. You can either focus on gentle pressure down towards the body and along the spine, or on drawing the energy up, depending on what you need to do. You don't need to use very strong physical pressure here because this is a powerful point that responds much better to a lighter energy focus.

Getting into position

You can practise neck work in a variety of
positions. The easiest one with which to start
is with the mother sitting the wrong way round
on a chair (but not if she has symphysis pubis
disorder), or on or leaning over a ball.

Stand or kneel beside her, and begin by
generally relaxing the mother's neck by cupping
the base of her skull with the "web" of one
hand – the area between the thumb and index
finger. Place the other hand over her forehead,
being careful not to cover her eyes, then gently
use that hand to ease her head back onto your
other hand. This won't be a huge movement,
but it creates a generalized pressure on the
base of her skull.

STROKING

You may want to use light hand-over-hand
stroking over her head and down her shoulders
to move energy and relax her. Experiment with
what feels more appropriate for her. Slower
strokes are generally more relaxing and faster
ones more stimulating.

You can carry the stroking down over her
whole back and onto her sacrum, and then
continue on down her legs.

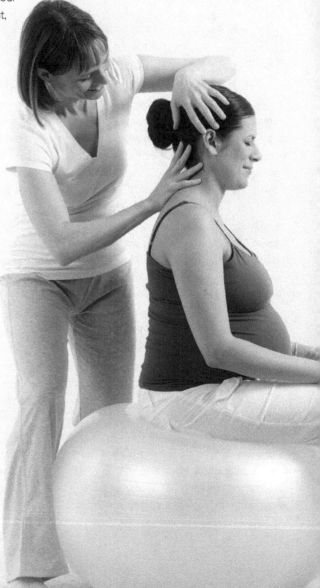

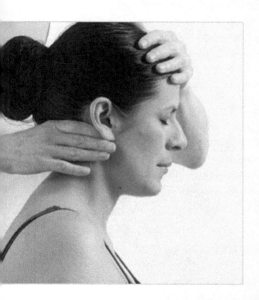

A mother will often enjoy having her partner work on her head during labour, especially if work on the sacrum is feeling too intense. Head work is often especially useful as a way to bring focus during transition, or during the second stage when the mother might not want so much work on the sacrum and abdomen.

SHOULDER LEANING

A good way of working the mother's shoulders is by using the technique of shoulder leaning to release tension or excess energy from the shoulder area, and also to provide you with an opportunity to rest your hands.

Simply place your forearms over the tops of the mother's shoulders and lean in the direction of her spine and down towards her feet. If you and she like, you also can do some stroking and rolling with your forearms to make the massage even more effective.

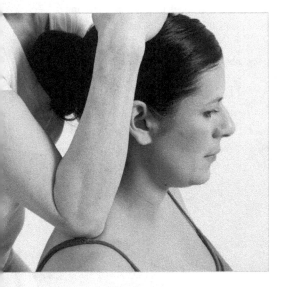

Shoulder leaning is often useful in transition and second stage, when the mother often holds tension in the shoulders. However, it is a useful technique to use at any time in labour if you notice that the mother is tightening her shoulders and jaw.

SHOULDER PRESSURE

You can combine this tension-releasing work with a shoulder massage, which is relaxing for the mother both during pregnancy and in labour. It involves putting pressure onto a point in the hollow on top of the shoulder, straight up from the nipple, which is in the highest point of the muscle on the shoulder. Do not practise this before 38 weeks, because the pressure points that it uses are powerful labour focus points (see page 78).

Place your thumbs directly in the GB21 points (see page 83) and lean down in the same way as for the general shoulder relaxing, or press down onto them with your elbows.

As with other labour focus points, pressure on these shoulder points will create a very strong downward effect. Using them may release tension in the neck and shoulders and release the jaw. They may help the baby to move downwards at any stage of labour, and are especially good for connecting with the downward contractions of second stage and feeling the movement of the baby coming down. They are also good for helping to deliver a retained placenta.

Shiatsu and massage for the

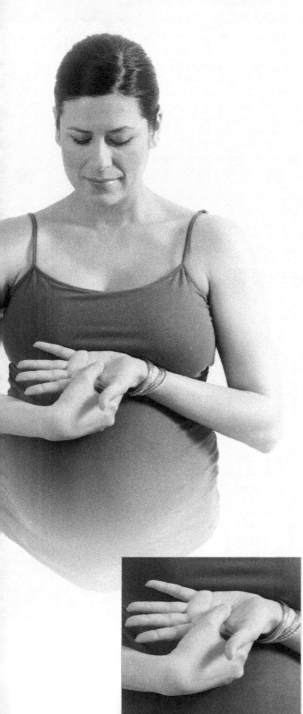

Sometimes, a mother will prefer having her arms and legs worked to having an all-body massage, which may sometimes feel too intense. Arm and leg work is generally less intimate and intrusive, and is a way of giving her a little more space.

OPENING YOUR HANDS

This can be a very beneficial exercise that the mother can do on her own. It massages the point in the centre of the palm known in shiatsu as Heart Protector 8 (HP8). Heart Protector 8 (HP8) is said to be the mirror of the Kidney 1 (K1) point on the feet (see page 77, picture 4). Linked with fire and the energy of the heart, this point helps to calm the emotions when you press it firmly but gently.

THE PRACTICE

Tighten your hands by clenching your fingers and drawing them to the centre of your palm. Notice what happens to your breathing and to your pelvis. Now open out your hands and relax them. Focus on the point in the centre of the palm and feel like you are breathing out through here. You can imagine that your hand is like a flower opening.

In this position you may enjoy pressure on the HP8. It is a useful point to work yourself or your partner can hold your hands with your fingers open and work the points.

arms and legs

ARM MASSAGE

You can give the mother an arm massage in any of the birthing positions. So before you begin, you need to find a comfortable position for yourself in which you can comfortably reach all the way from her shoulder to her hand. Depending on the position that she is in, you could stand sit or kneel,

THE PRACTICE

One easy arm massage technique involves simply gliding the palms of your hands up and down the mother's arms. Put your hands side by side on one of her wrists, with your fingers pointing towards her shoulder. Now slide the outside hand up to her shoulder and the other hand to her armpit, then slide them back down to her wrist. Repeat this as often as she wants, then massage her other arm in the same way.

You also could try a more powerful version of this basic stroke. Begin as before with both hands on her wrist, but as you glide them up her arm, press firmly but gently with your thumbs. Slide your hands up only as far as her elbow before bringing them down again to her wrist. Again, repeat this as often as the mother wants, then massage her other arm in the same way.

Whichever of these massage strokes you use, it can be nice to finish by holding the mother's hands and facing her. This may be very reassuring for her if she wants close contact with you, especially eye contact.

You can give her an arm massage at any time during pregnancy. When you finish and are holding her hands, focus on holding the HP8 point in the centre of each palm.

IN LABOUR

Arm massage and pressure on the HP8 points may be helpful if the mother is feeling panicky and uneasy. It also can be useful if she is not feeling comfortable in her environment or is feeling disconnected from her baby. At this point, holding her hands and looking into her eyes may be very comforting for her.

Pressure on the HP8 points or simply opening the hands also may be useful during labour for relieving anxiety, and for helping to open up the cervix. If the mother clenches her hands, this blocks the flow of energy to the rest of her body, including her cervix. Pain-distraction techniques that involve holding something sharp, like a comb, in one's hands are not a good idea from a shiatsu point of view because they involve restricting the flow of energy.

Holding her hands and looking into her eyes can be very comforting for her

LEG MASSAGE

You can give a leg massage with the mother in any of the birthing positions, but the simplest way to do it is with the mother standing and you kneeling next to her. Using a firm but gentle stroking movement, first down the outside and then up the inside of each leg, can stimulate her energy flows.

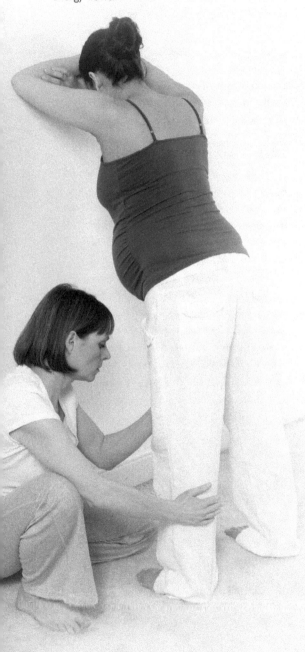

Meridian stroking technique

This massage stimulates all the shiatsu energy meridians in a mother's legs and is helpful in pregnancy for poor circulation, leg cramps and edema (but be a little cautious with this and focus on light strokes, particularly if the edema is fairly severe). Do not stroke directly over a varicose vein.

THE PRACTICE

Start with one hand at the top of a leg and one hand at the bottom. Vigorously stroke the top hand down the outside of the leg while at the same time moving the other hand up the inside of the leg. Keep the movement flowing while you lightly move the hands back to where they started. Repeat this as often as the mother wants, then massage her other leg in the same way.

IN LABOUR

Meridian stroking can be very useful during labour itself if the mother is feeling tired, and particularly if her legs are feeling wobbly. This is most likely to happen during transition.

FOOT MASSAGE

Simply holding a mother's feet can be very relaxing for her both in pregnancy and in labour. Many meridians start or end in the foot, and it important to have energy flowing through relaxed toes. If the toes are tight, then energy will not flow through them. You can feel the physical effects of this if you clench your toes and then you open them out. As you clench them you can probably feel that the leg muscles tighten as well as the pelvis and perineum. As you relax them, you feel everything else relaxing.

THE PRACTICE

With the mother in the all-fours position or leaning over a ball, stroke down her legs and finish by holding her feet. Then take one foot

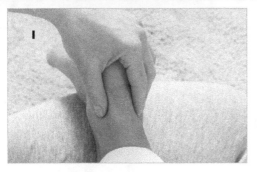

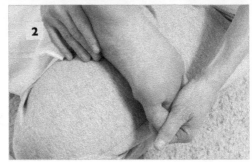

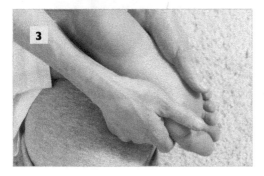

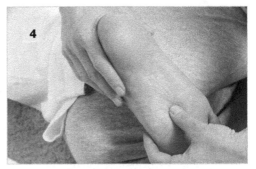

at a time and rest it over one of your thighs (1). You also can massage firmly over the top (2) and bottom of the foot, and stretch out the toes (3) and massage in between them.

While you are working on the feet, take the opportunity to stimulate the shiatsu pressure point that lies just below the centre of the ball of the foot, in a depression formed when the toes are curled (4). This point, known as Kidney 1 (K1) or the bubbling spring, is the lowest point on the body. When pressed, it is said to help the body absorb the Yin energy of the earth, so it is very calming.

IN LABOUR

Holding or working the feet in between contractions can often be very relaxing and help the mother to let go and rest.

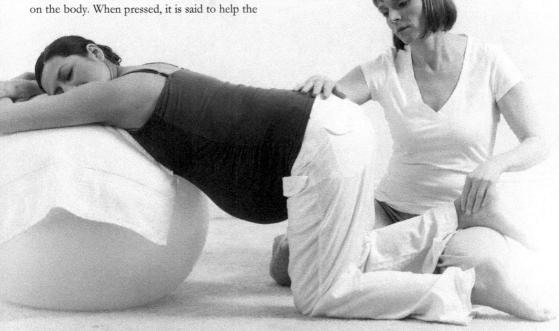

Labour focus points

There is a set of shiatsu points that, in women, have a strong effect on the uterus and the reproductive hormones. Some of these are "elimination" points, which are frequently stimulated outside pregnancy to treat headaches, sickness, cramp or constipation. They are often called the induction points, but I prefer to call them labour focus points because they don't work in the same way as labour-inducing drugs. When your birth partner stimulates your labour focus points for you, they will not make you go into labour if you are not ready, but they will help to release energy that can support you when you are. You also can use them during labour itself.

Provided you only use these points for as long and as often as they feel comfortable, then you cannot force yourself into labour before you are ready, or overstimulate the uterus and create overly strong contractions. However, they do help to ready your body for giving birth, and they do help the process of labour to flow. They also affect your baby, so they will help your baby to prepare for his birth. You can work them yourself if you prefer to be in your own space.

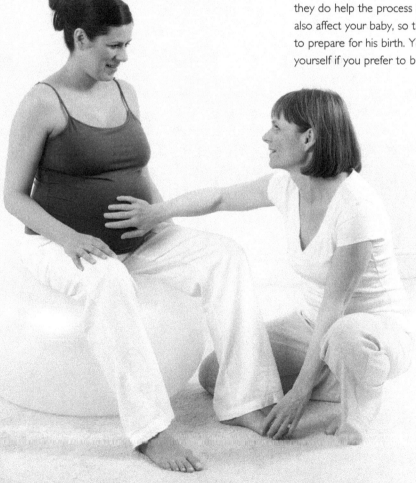

How they work

The labour focus points work by balancing energy in your body's meridians. They do not put anything into your body, they simply help what is already there to flow better. This means that they affect different people in different ways. Each point has a distinct effect and mothers will respond to those particular points, which produce the effects they need. As only some will work for you, you are not likely to need to use them all. If a point is a good one for you, you will probably know immediately because it will just "feel right". The point may help you to feel very relaxed, it may stimulate movement of your baby or it may even stimulate contractions.

When to use the points

Because many of the labour focus points are strong elimination points, they should not be stimulated during pregnancy before term (that is, before around 37-38 weeks).

If you use them at any stage in the late second and early third trimesters when your baby is fully developed, then they will probably have no effect because your body is not ready to give birth. However, if your body is trying to go into labour prematurely, stimulating the points may help your body to do so. While they won't create premature labour, they can help it along, so be especially wary of using them if you have a history of premature labour.

It is definitely not a good idea to use these points during the first trimester. when your body is trying to hold on to your baby and needs support to do that. Using the points will not create the miscarriage of a healthy baby, but they may encourage a body that is attempting to miscarry.

The labour focus points are useful from 37–38 weeks, because that is when your body and baby are preparing for birth. You can use them from this time on for as often as feels comfortable, but if they don't feel comfortable, then stop working them.

If your pregnancy is going overdue and medical induction is threatened, use them for as long and as often as you can, because their cumulative effect can be more powerful than using them just once. You also can try combining points – sometimes this is more effective than using individual ones. Be guided by your feelings when combining points; if they feel powerful, use them, but if they feel strange, don't. You are joining two different energies together, which may or may not be helpful.

These points help to focus your body and your baby on getting ready for labour, as well as supporting the process of labour itself

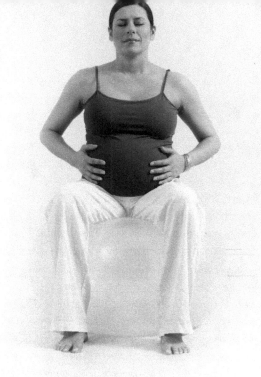

As "induction" points they are very effective. There are many reasons why mothers don't go into labour. For some mothers, fear or anxiety keeps them from going into labour, while others are simply too busy to focus on labour and haven't had the time to prepare. Still others enjoy being pregnant and don't want the experience to end.

Using the points helps by balancing both emotional and physical energies to encourage labour to begin.

Using the points in labour

Some mothers find some of these points helpful for pain relief during labour because they are allowing energy to flow. In labour, they can be used as long and as often as the mother wants, which could be for the whole of labour or for short periods only. A mother may just want one of the points to be held for hours, or she may want different points stimulated at different stages. I give indications of the effects of different points, but they are all potentially helpful at any stage of labour, both to help labour flow and to ease discomfort. The best way to use them is to try them out: you are not going to cause any harm by using the "wrong" point. That point will simply not feel right, so just stop using it and there will be no adverse effects. Often a mother will find that at least one of the points help her body to focus and get on with what it needs to do, and that's why I prefer to call them labour focus points.

As well as helping to focus your body and your baby on getting ready for labour, these points also support the process of labour itself. Because they don't put anything into your body and are simply working to balance your energy, you can use them alongside drugs if necessary, as there will be no interaction.

Locating and working the points

The following instructions are intended to guide the birth partner when giving shiatsu. Once you have found the point, it is often easiest to work into it with your thumb, but make sure that the rest of your hand is comfortable. It is often good to wrap the other fingers around the area you are working. You

Take notice!

Situations in which working the labour focus points can be especially useful:
- Preparing for labour
- get labour started when you are "overdue"
- to help move on a prolonged labour
- for pain relief during labour
- to strengthen ineffectual contractions
- to help deliver a retained placenta, or simply deliver a placenta without the use of drugs

Always remember: use the points as often and as long as feels right for you, but if they don't feel right, then stop using them.

can work both points at the same time – there is one on each limb – or you can work one point at a time. If you are working one point, place your free hand on another area of the mother's body where it feels comfortable and reassuring. Do what feels best for the mother, but do work both sides at some time, even if you work more one side than the other.

Try working the points in the different birth positions so you can feel comfortable and work out the best position for you. It really isn't possible to say how long you should work the points for because different mothers respond differently. However, you will probably need to work them for at least a minute to get an effect and be able to tell whether or not it is a good point to work.

Some mothers don't feel anything to start with and with these women, you have to hold the point for longer. However, if your partner continues to not feel anything, then either you are on the wrong point, so re-check the location, or you just need to keep holding for a little longer. If she still can't feel anything after a couple of minutes, then this probably isn't a point that is going to help her.

After some time, the mother will feel she has had enough. Before labour, this might be after just a few minutes, but if she is nearly ready to go into labour, then she might like to have it worked for as long as 20 minutes or more.

During labour, some mothers find they really do want the points held for hours. However, others may find that they don't want any more after 5 or 10 minutes, but then a few hours or minutes later, they want the point worked again.

PERINEAL MASSAGE

This is something that is not for everyone, but if you can do it, it will help you feel less self conscious about the stretching of your perineum in the second stage. Using massage to prepare your perineum for labour will not only ready it for the huge amount of stretching it has to do during labour but also help you to feel more connected and hopefully less afraid of what is going to happen.

You can begin to do this from about 32-34 weeks of pregnancy. You could even get your partner to do it. Do this ideally every day or so for at least a few minutes.

The exercise

- Lubricate your fingers well with oil. Any vegetable oil will be good, but do not use a petroleum-based oil.
- Rub enough oil onto the outside of the perineum to allow your fingers to move smoothly. The oil also feeds the skin and makes it more supple.
- Use your fingers to stretch out the perineum's skin in different directions: from the middle to the outside, up, down, and up and down together.
- Oil your index finger or your thumb thoroughly. You may need to try both to see which suits you best.
- Place your finger or thumb inside your vagina up to the second knuckle. Gently massage the vagina in a rhythmic U-shaped movement. This will gently stretch the vaginal tissues and muscles.
- When you are confident and comfortable, increase the pressure and introduce a stretch downwards. This should sting slightly – this same stinging sensation occurs when the baby's head is born.

Caution Do not do any perineal massage if you have vaginal herpes, thrush or any other vaginal infection. The massage could worsen and spread the infection.

WORKING THE LABOUR FOCUS POINTS

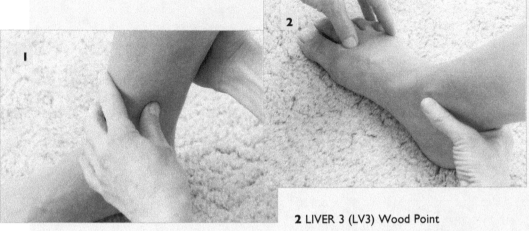

1 SPLEEN 6 (SP6) Earth Point

This point is often used by non-pregnant women for easing period pains because it regulates earth energies and has a strong effect on muscle tone. Earth, water and wood energies converge there, and these are all important elemental energies in labour.

Working this point may help change your baby's position and be useful for regulating uterine bleeding. It also has a strong toning and stimulating effect on the uterus. In Japan, it is often used on a regular basis during the whole of the last three months to strengthen the uterus. It really is worth trying this point at any stage of labour, as well as before it.

Place the tip of your little finger on top of the anklebone of the opposite leg, fingers pointing to the front of the leg. SP6 will then lie beneath the second joint of your forefinger, under the shin and three thumb-widths above the tip of the ankle bone.

2 LIVER 3 (LV3) Wood Point

The emotion associated with wood is anger; when emotions are suppressed, it is often wood energy that gets stuck. Working this point is very good for clearing blocked wood energy – either by bringing more energy into the body or by taking an excess away – and can help you release emotions and become more in touch with what you are feeling both before and during labour.

Suppressed emotions often may block going into labour as well as the movement from first to second stage labour, so this can be a good point to use during transition. It can, however, be used at any stage in labour and is also good to support the flow of wood energy in the second stage, so you can birth your baby. Working the point may help release tension in the shoulders and neck and so is helpful for headaches, which can be common in labour, and is often useful if the mother finds pressure on the neck and shoulder points too intense.

This point lies on top of the foot between the first and second toes, one-and-a-half to two thumb-widths back from the margin of the web.

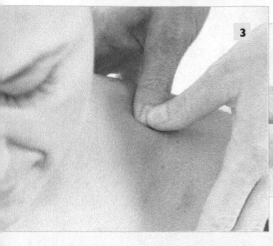

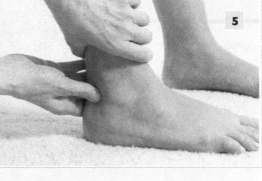

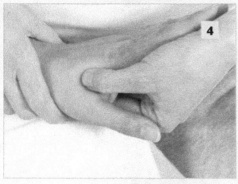

3 GALL BLADDER 21 (GB21) Wood Point

Pressure on this point can be incorporated into a shoulder massage to relax tension in the shoulder, neck and jaw and to help with the opening of the mouth and the perineum during second stage labour.

Because it seems to be linked with the release of oxytocin – the hormone involved in the third stage – this point is particularly good to help with the delivery of the placenta. Many midwives I have shown this point to have used it to avoid having to remove the placenta surgically, when it has refused to come out.

The point lies in the hollow on top of the shoulder, straight up from the nipple when you are standing. It is in the highest point of the muscle on the shoulder. An accurate way is to measure from the seventh cervical vertebra out along the neck.

4 LARGE INTESTINE 4 (LI4) Metal Point

This point is known as the "great eliminator" and is often used to relieve pain. This can be especially useful if the mother is feeling sick or has diarrhea, which is often the case leading up to labour, and even during labour itself. It also is good for headaches.

It is situated on the back of hand, between the thumb and forefinger. To locate it, have the thumb and index finger closed: the point is at the highest spot of the muscle.

Alternatively, stretch the thumb and the index finger. The point is then midway between the junction of the first and second finger bones and the border of the web, slightly towards the second finger bone.

5 BLADDER 60 (BL60) Fire & Water Point

The fire (heart) point on the bladder (water energy) meridian has the useful effect of clearing heat and excess energy, especially from the head. The point activates the whole length of the bladder meridian, so it can help ease any tightness in the head, spine and legs. It has a strong downward effect and is very useful for inducing and strengthening labour contractions, and for the expulsion of the placenta.

The point lies in the hollow midway between the knob of the anklebone on the outside of ankle and the outer Achilles tendon of the foot.

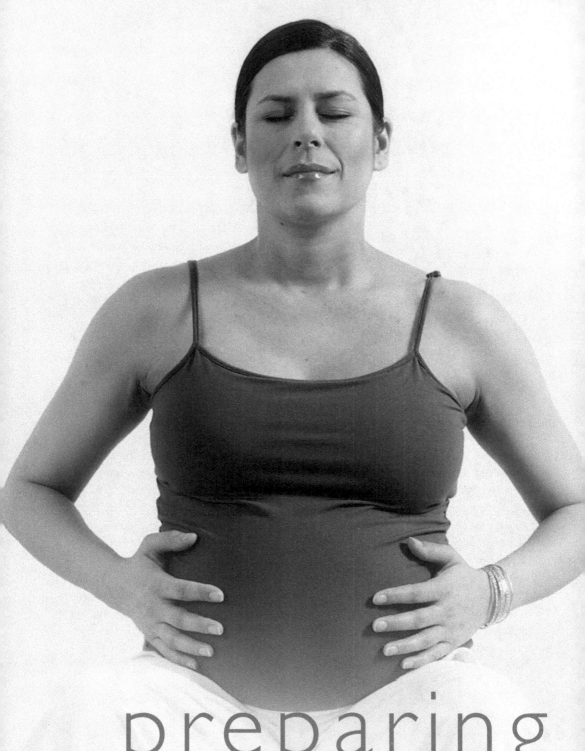

preparing

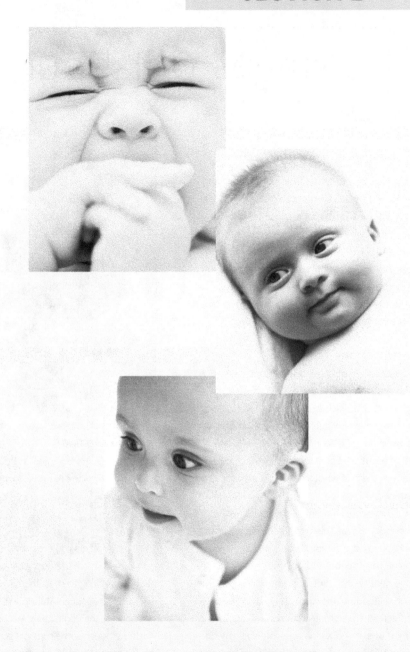

for birth

The stages of labour

The process of labour is usually thought of as having three different stages, but they are not always clearly defined for the mother and sometimes they flow into each other. Each stage has a different focus and it is useful to know what the stages are, but always remember that each mother experiences labour in a different way, and her experience of it may vary from one pregnancy to another. After the three stages of labour there also is a very important fourth stage – bonding with your baby.

Contractions

All three stages of labour are characterized by contractions, which are slightly different for each mother at each stage. Some mothers, for example, have very intense contractions right at the beginning of labour, while others feel only slight discomfort, Some women may not even be aware of them at all, other than their abdomens hardening.

What happens during a contraction is that your abdomen and uterus tighten. In early labour, this happens at the top of your uterus – similar to tightening a belt. As labour progresses, the movement becomes more rhythmical and co-ordinated until the whole of your uterus is contracting. Those mothers who are very aware of their uterus and abdomen tightening may or may not find it painful; others may feel pain from the contractions referred down into their back or their legs.

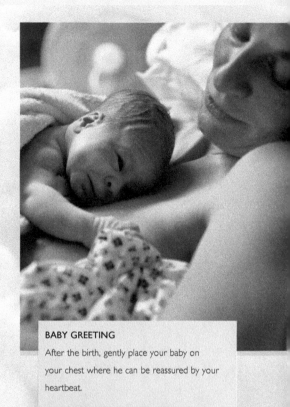

BABY GREETING
After the birth, gently place your baby on your chest where he can be reassured by your heartbeat.

Most mothers find the most helpful thing to do is to work with the feelings of each contraction, rather than trying to resist them.
In a labour that starts naturally, that is, one that is not induced, the contractions will usually start quite weakly, although some mothers go straight into intense contractions. Contractions are like waves in that they build up in the body to reach a peak

Go with the feelings of each contraction, rather than trying to resist them – you even may find you enjoy them

of intensity and then fade away gradually. The body usually has time – even if it is only 30 seconds – to get used to each contraction before it reaches its greatest intensity. It helps to start focusing on a contraction when it is beginning, so that its peak doesn't take you by surprise and to use the space in between to rest and prepare for the next one. This will help to prevent tiredness and conserve energy.

An induced labour tends to be harder because the contractions are less like waves and more intense, constant and contracting. There is not the same kind of build-up to the intensity at the peak of a contraction, nor the rest in between. Some mothers work with these contractions without pain-killing medication, but they require more focus.

Waters can break at any stage of birth, and sometimes not at all. If they break before birth begins, there is a potential risk of infection, so you will be monitored and perhaps induction suggested after a time frame: then it can be useful to use the points to support labour to begin. Often they break at the end of first stage and support the movement of the baby out. Sometimes they don't break at all. Waters help protect the baby from the power of the contractions.

PAIN RELIEF TECHNIQUES

Breathing/Visualizations

Some mothers find that focusing on something else, such as an external object or a number, may help block out pain. However, most mothers find it is more helpful to use something related to what the contraction is doing. This mental image could be a wave in the first stage or a bulb pushing through the ground for the second stage. It is important to spend time exploring in advance what you think might be likely to work for you. As contractions are like waves, such visualizations are often the most helpful.

Positions

Moving around and assuming different postures tends to help ease any discomfort or pain. Using the resting versions of the birth positions (see pages 30-39) to relax between contractions will help conserve energy.

Massage

Some mothers find that certain touch techniques help their contractions to be more effective and less painful, or less frightening. As labour progresses, you will find that you will get into a rhythm, which will be your rhythm of labour. Labour is very similar to a dance; you just need to find the right step and rhythm, and then you are on your way.

First stage labour

The first stage is the phase of labour that takes the longest and can vary most in length of time. It is divided into the latent phase, when the opening of the cervix dilates (widens) to up to 3 cm, and the active phase, when the cervix dilation increases from 3 cm to 10 cm.

It is often hard to know whether labour really has begun or not. Some mothers seem to have quite long latent first stages, while others go straight into active labour.

The latent phase of the first stage can last for days with irregular contractions, or may even pass unnoticed. It is sometimes known as the "stop/start" phase of labour, because the contractions don't get progressively stronger and closer together but are rather more sporadic. There can be an hour or two of quite strong and frequent contractions, which can be quite painful, especially if the baby is in the posterior position, but which then stop. These contractions usually last about 30-40 seconds each, and the intervals between them can vary from about 3 minutes to 20 minutes. What is happening is that the uterus is contracting but the contractions are not co-ordinated. Some practitioners call them "warm-up" contractions. Sometimes, if your baby is not in the best position for birth, your uterus is contracting to help her change position rather than to dilate the cervix.

The active phase usually lasts around 10-12 hours, but it can last for as little as 1 hour or as much as 36 hours or more. The contractions get stronger and closer together, lasting for at least 40 seconds, and happen every 3-4 minutes.

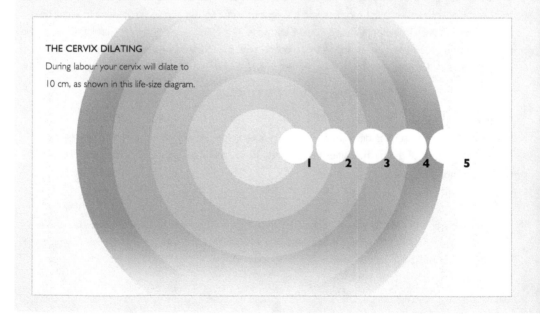

THE CERVIX DILATING

During labour your cervix will dilate to 10 cm, as shown in this life-size diagram.

1   2   3   4   5

Slowed progress

The progress of the first stage of labour can sometimes be slowed, or even blocked, for a variety of reasons including fear and anxiety, lying on your back, exhaustion and lack of food.

If you are at all fearful or anxious about going into labour, these feelings will increase the amount of the hormone adrenaline flowing in your bloodstream. Adrenaline inhibits the production of endorphins and oxytocin, your body's natural pain killers, so labour becomes more painful. The release of adrenaline is part of the body's "fight and flight" mechanism. If you feels "threatened" during labour, you may either give birth quickly or stop giving birth altogether. Labour often stops, therefore, when a mother moves from home to hospital because the mother is leaving her "safe" space to enter a new, and possibly quite intimidating, place and she may feel threatened. (Some mothers, however, find being in hospital reassuring.) This is why it is so helpful to have a safe space to go to if you are giving birth in hospital, whether it be a space visualized in your mind or one created by taking a favourite and reassuring object in with you.

You will feel your abdomen hardening, as you may have done in latent first stage; this is your uterus contracting. Contractions will occur more rhythmically and strongly as first stage progresses, and labour will be considered established. In this stage, your baby's bottom, which hopefully is at the top of the uterus, is being pressed down, so the head pushes deeper into your pelvis. The pressure of the head stimulates your perineum, which in turn brings about stronger contractions.

BREATHING

Most women find that breathing in a rhythm that feels natural to them is most helpful. It could include making a sound or simply breathing out.

KEEP FOCUSED

Encouragement from your birth partner and attendants is vital to maintaining your focus and attention. Everyone needs to keep positive and relaxed, whatever is going on.

I have seen many mothers doing fine in labour and then just one misplaced comment from someone around them, such as "Are you sure you don't want that epidural?", makes them question what they are doing and how they are coping. It is amazing how, from one minute to the next, a labouring moher can go from being incredibly focused and coping exceedingly well to not being able to cope at all.

POSITIONS

Use the positions outlined in "the fundamentals" and identify the most comfortable; you may move a lot or stay still.

Lying on your back and being immobile tends to make labour more painful because your baby is compressed against your back. There also is less space for the baby to move and gravity is not helping her to move down, so your labour is slowed. Try to avoid lying immobile on your back for any length of time, but don't think you have to be active from the moment you have a contraction. It is so important to rest and do the minimum.

If you have a long labour, you will get exhausted moving around for hours and hours. Exhaustion will slow your labour down because as you get tired, so does your uterus.

MASSAGE
At some point you may feel you need extra support from your partner, perhaps in the form of a massage. Using different massage techniques, on whatever area of your body you need them, will often help you to relax. The most helpful area to massage is usually the lower back, but massaging any other area, including the hands and feet, can be beneficial.

Sometimes, mothers like different areas of their body worked more during contractions than in between the contractions.

Of course, if you go into active labour in the middle of the night and you need your partner to support you, either emotionally or in different positions or by giving you massage, then go with whatever works best.

PROPER NOURISHMENT
Because labour can be long, it is important to eat and drink as and when you feel like it. Imagine going without food for more than 24 hours

How you can help your body

As the first stage of labour can last so long, and you don't know how long it is going to last, it is very important that both you and your partner conserve your energies. The best way to do this is for both of you to do the minimum you need at any given time, and to use the space between contractions to really let go and rest. This is even more important if you go into labour in the middle of the night, because if you miss out on your sleep, you are going to get even more tired.

Doing the minimum usually means beginning with the breathing and visualization techniques so that you and your baby are getting enough oxygen. If this is all you need, then let your body, and your partner, rest.

By breathing deeply, you help your body produce endorphins and oxytocin, which are its natural pain killers. Of course, being relaxed in labour is not the same kind of relaxation as when you are practising the breathing techniques. You will be using the same kind

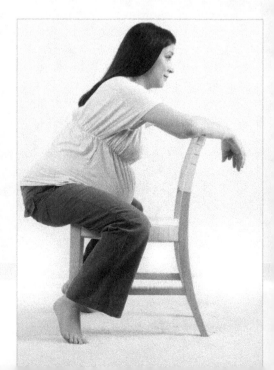

and working hard without even being pregnant, and then think how much more difficult that would be when you are nourishing a baby as well.

Some mothers don't feel like eating or feel sick after eating, but if you feel like eating, eat and drink whatever you want. You need to keep energy coming into your body because you are using up a lot through the contractions. If you don't feel

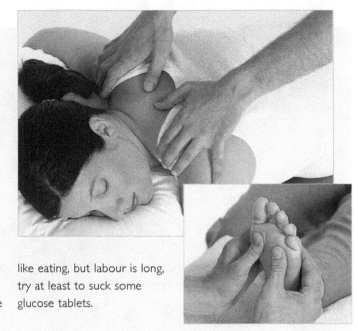

like eating, but labour is long, try at least to suck some glucose tablets.

of techniques, but from the outside you may not look at all relaxed in the conventional way because you could be moving or making noises. Being relaxed in labour means allowing your body to get on with what it needs to, without resisting. Use whatever breathing, sounds or visualizations seem most helpful.

Being in a comfortable position will help you feel more relaxed. It could be one position, or combinations of different positions. You could be moving a lot or you could be still. Use whatever works for you.

If you do need to move around, then do so, but if you are comfortable lying down, then do so, using comfortable resting positions such as side-lying or forward leaning. If you are moving, use resting positions, such leaning over a ball, as much as you can.

The best positions are those that allow your pelvis and baby to move. These will help labour to progress well and also to be less painful, and could be simply lying on your side or resting. Upright positions in which you are leaning forward and not compressing your pelvis tend to help labour progress the most, and gravity will help your baby move down. Leaning forward will help keep your pelvis open so that your baby can move and not get stuck, and take the pressure away from your lower back, relieving tension here. If you are mobile, that will further support this process of opening up your hips and pelvis and allowing the baby to move. If you have practised these positions in advance, they will feel quite intuitive and you will quickly find the right ones to use.

Transition

At the end of the first stage of labour, you go through a phase called transition, in which your body begins to get ready for the second stage.

In transition, your cervix completes its final stages of dilation, from 8 cm to 10 cm, and your contractions are closer together. They will come maybe every two minutes and also will be longer, lasting for up to 60 seconds.

Physically, everything gets more intense. You may feel hot and then cold, have shaky legs, feel nauseous, grunt, feel pressure in your anus or empty your bowels. Emotionally, it also can get very intense. You may get angry and feel you can't go on. You may shout at your partner or ask for an epidural or Caesarean, even though you have been doing fine up to now.

Transition may be brief, just a few minutes, or it may last a while, up to an hour or more. The important thing for both you and your partner to remember is that all of this intensity shows that your body is getting on with labour and preparing to give birth. It means that things are moving on. If you can see all the effects of transition as good signs and accept them, you will

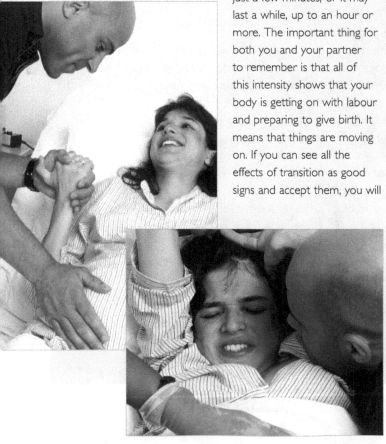

find it much easier to cope. You may feel an urge to push because of the pressure of your baby's head pushing down more, but this can sometimes happen before your cervix is completely dilated. It is usually best to try and hold back from pushing as much as you can. If it is impossible to stop, then it is probably time to push, but often a mother will start trying to push because she feels that is what should happen next. However, pushing isn't about forcing a baby out, but letting the body give birth.

It is important to wait until you feel strong second-stage contractions before bearing down, because your baby may still need to adjust her position and bearing down may force her into the wrong position.

Sometimes there can be a pause when the cervix is fully dilated. Some mothers feel like going to sleep then, especially if it has been a long first stage. Some midwives call this the "rest and be thankful" stage. It makes sense for your body to have a little rest before going into the potentially more physically demanding second stage.

Slowed progress

As with first stage, there are a number of factors that can slow or block the progress of transition. These include fear and anxiety, feeling unheard, exhaustion, giving up, being in any uncomfortable position, and lying on your back, which compresses your sacrum and makes the whole process more painful.

How you can help your body

Staying relaxed and focused in whatever way helps you will support this stage of labour. You still need to focus on your breathing and on relaxing, but you also need to have more of a focus down into your perineum. Perineal massage (see page 81) will help you to connect with it.

Use positions where gravity helps, but make sure that you are relaxing as much as you can in them rather than forcing things to happen. If anything, it is better to try to wait, to control and hold back slightly until you feel you need to get into the pushing of the second stage.

You may or may not want to be touched during transition, but it is possible that massage will help release tension from stressed areas of your body. Often, at this stage, the pressure on your sacrum becomes extremely intense and you may need more pressure when your partner massages it. Your legs may become shaky, so massage to stimulate them may be helpful, and if you find yourself losing connection with yourself, your breathing and your baby, some holding work on your abdomen could be useful. Or you may simply need your partner to hold the calming points of your hands or feet.

Pushing isn't about forcing the baby out, but letting the body give birth

Second stage labour

This is the stage in which your baby is born, and you experience expulsive contractions, which work to move your baby down the birth canal and out into the world.

It is important that you do not push unless you really feel the urge to, because your baby may still need to make some final shifts and turns and could get stuck if you try to force her out.

Like all the stages of labour, the second stage can vary greatly from one woman to another, and from one pregnancy to the next. Some mothers don't need to bear down strongly and the baby comes out gently, but others have very strong contractions. Some babies are born within one or two contractions, while others take their time. However, it is usually best to try

to be patient, and hold back a little until the desire to push is overwhelming. Let your body take over, then go naturally with what you feel.

The bones of your pelvis are able to move to allow the birth process to happen and give enough space for your baby. Your coccyx actually moves slightly out of the way. It is important to realize that your bones can move, they are not fixed, and the more you can allow them to move, the easier second stage will be.

Your baby's head gradually comes down, and when it finally appears and can be seen, this is what is known as "crowning". At this point it is important not to suddenly push hard, because you can overstretch your perineum and increase your chances of tearing. You also will be forcing your baby out in a

more sudden way, which may cause more trauma for her.

Some babies come out quickly after crowning, but some seem quite happy to wait at the perineum and ease their way out. You may feel that you want to reach down and feel your baby's head. Some mothers find that this helps them to focus, but not all mothers will want to do this. Your partner may want to see the head, but shouldn't be worried if it looks blue – babies are very often quite blue when they are born.

This stage is shorter than first stage, and you will probably not be bearing down actively for more than about two hours, and perhaps for only about 15 minutes or even less if you've had a baby before. Take your time, there is no rush. Your baby will come when she is ready.

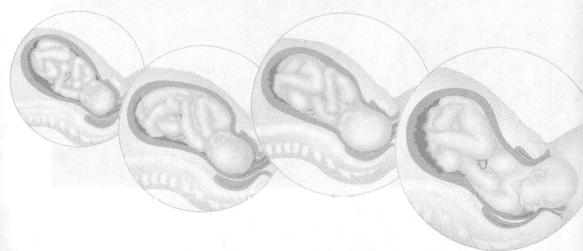

Slowed progress

The progress of second stage labour often can be slowed or blocked if you are over-anxious and trying to make it happen. You get very tense in your neck and shoulders, which means that there is a lot of pushing and effort going on but it is not very productive because all the focus is on your upper body. All this straining can be very tiring and you may find that you run out of energy.

Lying down on your back also often results in unproductive pushing, because it is harder to push up hill. Your baby is also more likely to get stuck because your pelvis is compressed and so the bones can't move so easily.

How you can help your body

Stay relaxed and don't panic, and stay focused on your breathing. Some mothers may find they don't want as much massage in this stage of labour, but others may find that it helps them to stay relaxed and focused. A good area to focus on with the massage is the neck and shoulders, which are often tense.

This stage is often portrayed as difficult and as though you have to push and strain, but, in fact, your baby will be born more easily if you don't push and strain. See it as working with your baby. Be patient, and just allow your baby to be born. Your body and your baby know what to do.

You need to focus on feeling your baby coming down onto your perineum and on going with the feelings of pressure. If you can, visualize your perineum stretching open. This is where perineal massage again comes in handy, and some mothers find it helpful to focus on something that helps them visualize the baby coming down, such as pulling down on a rope.

You should continue to use the upright positions to help your baby come down and also to widen your pelvic outlet, but you may need to use them in a more physical way. The standing squat can be particularly useful at this stage if you feel unsure about what to do.

Throughout the second stage, keep on doing whatever is working for you. Stay focused, using whatever breathing and visualizations work. You will find that the positions you prefer will vary, and you still need to rest between contractions. You also may find that you want to be in your own space and do not need so much massage or physical touch. Finally, be prepared to be taken over by the power of your baby coming down the birth canal.

Third stage labour

This is the stage in which you deliver the placenta; it is similar to the second stage but not nearly as intense. The placenta is much smaller than the baby and doesn't have any bones, so it is a lot easier to deliver through the passage already created by the bigger baby. The placenta is usually delivered with one contraction, sometimes almost straight after the baby, sometimes within 10-15 minutes and usually within an hour.

This stage is potentially dangerous, however, because if the blood vessels that attached the placenta to the wall of the uterus don't close up, there is a risk of haemorrhage. But if you have had a straightforward labour up to this point, without any heavy blood loss, you can continue with a natural approach. Your body is designed to deliver the placenta as well as the baby.

If you do start bleeding heavily, you will be given drugs that help contract the uterus and get the placenta out more quickly.

Slowed progress

If delivery of the placenta is delayed, it might be because you are not relaxed or are not in an upright position. It also could be because your bladder is full, or because you are exhausted.

How you can help your body

During third stage, a key element again is to stay relaxed and in touch with your body and your baby. If you want to deliver the placenta naturally, without using any drugs, you need to stay focused and in an upright position, but although this won't be as intense as second stage you probably won't feel like squatting.

If you have a full bladder, this can interfere with the delivery of the placenta so you may need to empty it, even if that is the last thing you feel like doing. Another way to encourage delivery is to breastfeed your baby. Breastfeeding stimulates the release of the hormone oxytocin into your bloodstream. This hormone helps the uterus to contract and deliver the placenta.

Fourth stage labour

Now all the work is done and you can just focus on deepening your connection with your baby. It is the beginning of the next phase in the journey of being a mother – becoming a family, getting to know your baby and accepting him as a separate being from you, outside the safety and protection of your womb.

The time immediately after birth, sometimes called "the golden hour", is a crucial period. If you have not had any drugs, then both you and your baby will be in a state of heightened sensitivity. It is the time to fall in love with your baby, who will begin feeding at your breast.

It can be a wonderful time for both parents to try to see things from their baby's perspective. He has been in the womb, which is quite a dark environment, for nine months. It was a bit of a shock for him to come out of the water, where he was completely supported, and into the air. Be with him and support him in this process of adjustment. Use your relaxation skills for the rest of your life together with your family, not just for the moment of birth.

Slowed progress

Having drugs, especially pethidine, blocks the process of bonding with your baby, as does having your baby taken away unnecessarily.

How you can help yourself

If you have had lots of support people with you during labour, this is the time for them to stand back and just allow you and the baby's father or your partner to be with your baby.

Essentially, however, what you need now is to have time and space in an environment that you feel is right for you and your baby. You might want to go back to your special place and see how your newborn baby fits into the space.

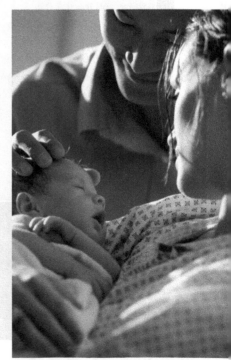

Working with pain

What most mothers and birth partners are worried about – not surprisingly, given our culture's usual portrayal of birth – is the pain. Most mothers feel pain at some times in labour – when the contractions become stronger or the pressure increases as the baby comes down the birth canal, for example. The pain is usually there for a purpose; it will prompt you to move or change your focus, or warns you that things aren't going so well. Even though pain may be present, you need to remember that your body is designed to be able to work with it.

A lot of the pain that women experience in labour is due to being afraid and fearful and therefore tense. Tension will tend to increase

Techniques to transform the pain

You can make labour much more bearable by using techniques such as breathing and visualization, changing your position, and massage and touch.

Just breathing out the discomfort often helps you to let it go. For example, if you feel sick, then breathing out the feelings of sickness and breathing in new energy will help. When you feel pain you often tense

more into it, which usually makes it worse, so breathing out helps you let go of the tension. You also might find that visualizing the pain as something – a colour, demon, prickly cactus or anything else that suits you – and then letting it go, helps relieve the pain.

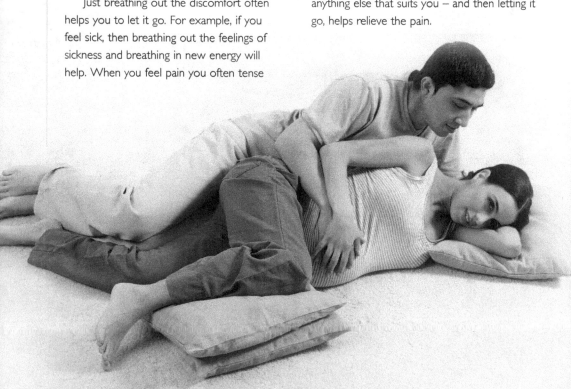

pain, so the more relaxed you are the less pain you will feel, because your body will produce more endorphins and oxytocin. The more anxious you are, the harder it is to cope with the pain. Resistance to pain, too, often creates more of it so acceptance is important in dealing with pain. First accept the pain, and then in doing so let it go.

Tiredness is another key factor. The more tired you are, the harder it is to cope with anything, especially pain.

Pain is also an issue for partners to explore. The mother may be coping well but the partner may get distressed and want to try to take the pain away. It is important for your partner to consider how he is going to react

Tension caused by pain often makes sufferers feel they need to curl up or lie down to relieve it. Because labour pain is quite specific, however, the positions for dealing with it also are quite specific and that is why I recommend practising the different ones. Use whichever of them work best for you.

Touch also can help to relieve labour pains; simply rubbing or massaging your abdomen, neck or back, or getting your partner to do it for you, can be soothing and relieve discomfort. In labour, there often are specific areas that are more in pain and these may need more or less touching.

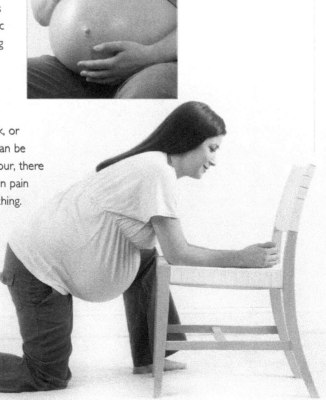

to seeing you in pain and the feelings that this may create in him. He needs to be careful not to impose what he thinks is right for you in terms of pain relief, if it is not what you want.

A big part of dealing with the pain of labour is about your belief in yourself. If you believe you can cope with it and focus on one contraction at a time, you usually can. If you start thinking it is all too much and you can't carry on, then it is easy to give up, and once you give up, everything starts to overwhelm you. Again, your birth partner has a vital role to play as key supporter. He needs to believe in you and what you are doing, and to encourage you in appropriate ways so that you don't give up.

Of course, sometimes the pain of labour is particularly intense and then your partner needs to be able to recognize that you really can't cope. For example, intense pain can be caused by the baby getting stuck in the wrong position. In that case the pain is a signal that something is not quite working properly, and this should be investigated.

The pain test

Although we can never re-create the pains of labour, which are unlike most other kinds of pain, we can get some idea of how we respond to pain and what things help us to cope better with it. This exercise is designed to help you and your birth partner explore your reactions to it, and learn how your partner might cope with seeing you in pain. It was devised by Pam England, founder of the Birthing from Within organization.

To start off, you and your partner each hold an ice cube for two minutes and note your reactions to it. Do you tense up? Which parts of your bodies become tense? How do you feel? Now you should hold another ice cube for a further two minutes

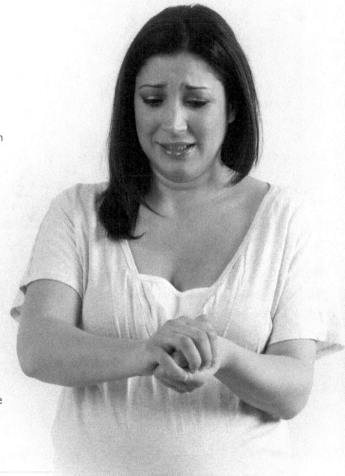

If the pain is really so bad that you feel you can't cope with it, there are drugs that will relieve it and sometimes they become necessary. During a long, difficult labour, drugs can help take the edge off things for a while and help you relax, making the rest of labour more bearable. You have to remember, however, that drugs aren't always 100 per cent effective and that all drugs will have some kind of side effect on both you and your baby.

Drugs do have a place in labour, but unfortunately they are often over-used. Do read books or talk to your midwife about the pros and cons of different drugs and interventions.

Usually, when you feel pain it is because something is wrong with your body. but in labour the pain is simply because your body is doing something that it may never have done before, and won't do very often. Labour does place huge intense physical and emotional demands on your body but, unless there are complications, it can deal with it.

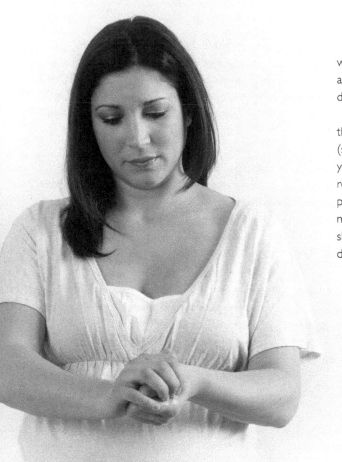

while your partner watches you and notes his responses to your discomfort.

It is a good idea to read through the relaxation section (see overleaf), and use what you've learned that helps you relax while you try the second part of the test again. What was most helpful with the ice cube should prove to be most helpful during labour.

Using relaxation

Relaxation is the main key to enjoying your baby's birth day, because by being relaxed, you give your body space to get on with labour. Your labour is actually less likely to be painful and your baby is less likely to become distressed.

Whatever it is that usually helps you feel relaxed in stressful situations will give you a clue as to what may help you relax in labour. A key role for your partner is to know how you are when you are relaxed, what helps you to relax and how to

Learning what works

You and your partner should make yourselves comfortable in a quiet space and close your eyes, if that feels the right thing to do. Breathe out slowly and deeply. With each out breath feel your body becoming more relaxed and at ease. You may choose to visualize your special space (see page 106) to do this. When you feel completely relaxed, focus on the following questions. Explore each question slowly and at some length. Notice if your breathing changes in any way.

- Do I find that music helps me relax, or is silence better? Or some of both?
- Do I find it more relaxing having people around me or being on my own?
- Do I relax more when I am moving around or being still?
- Do I relax more when I am outside or indoors?
- Do I find it more relaxing to focus on myself or on objects outside myself?
- Do I find being touched or massaged more relaxing than having some space?

- Which of the elements do I find most relaxing? Water? Water in the form of a gentle stream, a waterfall, the sea or a lake? Fire? A raging fire or a candle? Metal? A crystal or the out breath. Wood? A growing plant or a sturdy tree trunk? Earth? A tilled field or a sandy beach?

Explore these different questions from your state of relaxation. You will probably find that certain things are relaxing for you at particular times, but in different situations they are not.

Now the mother can try to imagine that she is giving birth, or the partner try to imagine he is watching his partner give birth. The mother should try to see herself experiencing a contraction and imagine feeling the pressure of the baby coming down deeper into her pelvis. She should try to think about the kind of things that could help her to relax during labour itself. Are they physical objects, are they thoughts, or are they positions in which she feels comfortable? Is it being touched or held in a particular way that would work? Is it music or is it silence? Is it people being around or being

support it. It is crucial that your partner is also relaxed, because being with someone who is not relaxed will itself create stress. It is not very convincing if your partner is telling you to relax and saying encouraging things if he is tense himself.

iIt is therefore important that both you and your partner read through the following section to explore your potential for relaxation.

on her own? Is it a particular element? Is it moving around or staying still? She should explore her different feelings and thoughts about being relaxed in labour.

For the partner, he can explore how he might feel watching the mother in labour. What feelings does it bring up for him? He also can think about how he might be able to feel more relaxed in his role as the observer of labour.

After a while, allow yourselves to come back to your bodies. Be aware of your breathing and follow the movement of your breath as you breathe out and in. Be aware of the way you are sitting or lying, and of how relaxed you are feeling. Gradually ease yourself back to where you are now and become aware of the space in which you are resting. On an out breath, open your eyes. Afterwards, discuss your different experiences.

Creating your birth space

The surroundings in which you give birth are very important. You may not have thought that much about your birth environment beyond whether you want to give birth at home or in hospital. However, regardless of where you choose to give birth, you can to some extent create your own space within it. You also can learn to connect with an imaginary space by focusing in on yourself. This may be helpful if you can't create the external space you want.

In her book *Rediscovering Birth*, Sheila Kitzinger describes how in many cultures in the past, birth would take place outside, where mothers were intimately connected with nature. Often they would have special shelters built for them outdoors. Slave mothers in the Caribbean would give birth next to the "birth tree" on the sugar plantation, Australian Aborigine mothers on a carpet of soft gum leaves, and New Guinean mothers on a bed of creepers.

Even today, some mothers choose to give birth outside. Russian mothers have been giving birth in the Black sea in the summer.

In some cultures, the birth space was a special or sacred space. In South Africa, for example, it would have been the mother's or father's grandmother's house, because it was considered the abode of the ancestors who would bless the birth. Zulu mothers gave birth in a hut decorated with precious objects as they believed the first things a baby saw must be beautiful.

We have strayed very far from this ideal. Now we tend to think more of safety and having the right equipment present, as in a hospital, during childbirth. But where do you want your baby's birth day party to take place? Would you feel comfortable about giving birth at home, with all your things around you or would you feel anxious in case something happened? Does a hospital reassure you or make you more anxious?

Hospital birth is really only necessary if things go wrong, but if you feel more at ease in a hospital, it is worth thinking about what sort of objects you might bring to make it beautiful for you and your baby. You can surround yourself with objects, either of a practical nature such as a comfortable mat or a soft, cuddly blanket, or that hold a special meaning for you such as a necklace, stone or picture. Some mothers find that they can create their ideal environment simply by imagining it, by going inside themselves and creating it in their minds. They don't

You can surround yourself with special objects, either of a practical nature… or items that hold a special meaning for you…

necessarily need the physical environment to support them.

If you are going to have your baby at home, it is much easier to create your ideal environment because it is your own space. Midwives and doctors have to ask to come in. It is more difficult in hospital because you are going into the midwives' and doctors' space. However, even in a hospital it is important to remember that the environment is there to support you. If you don't want the bed to be a certain height, if you want the lights dimmed or if you want pieces of medical equipment moved out of your way, you need to make sure it happens. Helping to get things the way you want them is a key part of your partner's role. Remember – it is your unique birth.

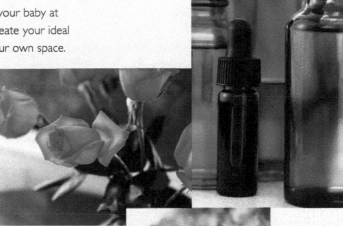

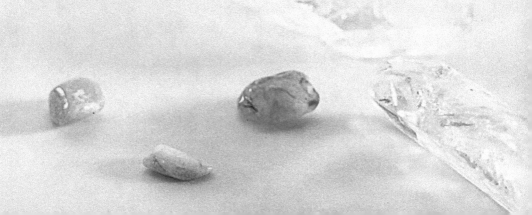

Special objects
Flowers, crystals and oils can all have a calming effect.

Visualizing your special birth place

The following exercise is designed to help you envisage how you want your birthing environment to be.

Sit or lie down in a comfortable space and relax your body. Close your eyes, if that feels the right thing to do. Breathe out slowly and deeply, and with each out breath feel your body becoming more relaxed and at ease. When you feel completely relaxed, begin imagining your ideal environment. What is the space in which you feel most comfortable? It could be a special place you love to go – a room in your house or somewhere else in a building, or an imaginary place or somewhere from a dream. Fully experience this special place.

Explore the first images that come to you. You could be in a forest or by a stream, on a sun-drenched beach or in a special place that you knew as a child. Let your imagination run away with you. Picture this place clearly in your mind. Look at the

different colours of your surroundings and any objects around you. Feel and interact with your environment. Is the sand coarse or rough? Do you feel water? Is it hot or cold? Evoke the smells and tastes.

Think about the five elements of earth, fire, water, metal and wood, and which of them are in your special place. Take time to explore each of these elements in turn. Notice which are present and any that are absent, and interact with each one you find there.

Immerse yourself fully in this environment and explore your feelings as you explore it. How do you see yourself in this space? What are you doing? Take some time to move within it and some time to be still and reflective.

From within this space, imagine the kind of place in which you would like to give birth. What sort of things do you want around you while you are giving birth? How do you see your body moving in this birth environment? What sort of images come to you now as you imagine

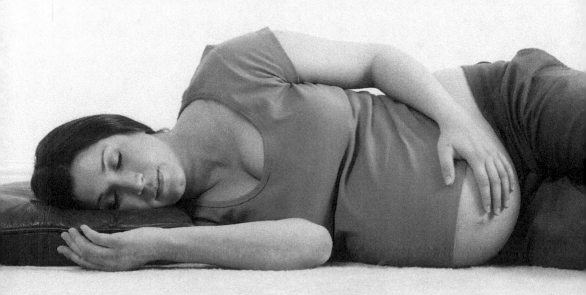

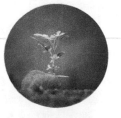

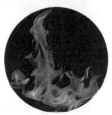

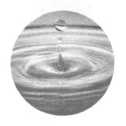

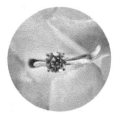

yourself giving birth to your baby?

Spend as long as you need to in your special space, then allow yourself to come back to your body. Be aware of your breathing, and follow the movement of your breath as you breathe in and out. Be aware of the way you are sitting or lying, and of how you are feeling in this moment. On an out-breath, open your eyes.

MAKING YOUR SPECIAL PLACE A REALITY

Now think about what you might take from your special place to have within your real birth environment. Think about how you can recreate as much of your visualization as possible with the options that you have. For example, if you feel you want to be by a running stream, it might be appropriate to think about a water birth.

Maybe you want to be by a warm fire, in which case home might be your best choice.

Or maybe you would feel more comfortable in hospital with medical equipment around you. If you plan on going to hospital, you might want to practise creating a more magical space to go to within your mind.

Write down descriptions of both your imagined birthing environment and your actual one. You could make a tape or journal of your imagined environment, to help to keep it real in your mind. You could then play the tape over to yourself, or read your journal in the days and weeks before your birth to keep this environment alive in your mind. Try to find some important words, thoughts or images that help you to find the key to your special place, and make a list of the things that you need to make your real environment the way you want it.

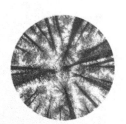

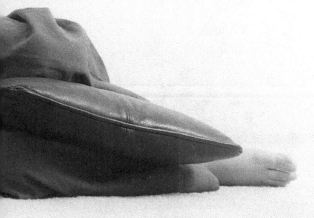

Choosing your birth partne

It is your baby's birth day – whom do you want at the party? Who is going to be in your environment? It is up to you to choose.

Your birth partner should be the person with whom you feel most able to be yourself, the one with whom you are relaxed and comfortable. You even can think about your birth partner in terms of elements: if he or she were an element, what would it be – a still stream? a fiery furnace? a rooted tree? Which of these elements do you feel you want in your space? This may influence your choice of birth partner, or make it clear to you whether you want only one partner or more than one.

Your birth partner also should want to be there. It is good to practise the different aspects of the birth preparation (breath, positions and massage) with your partner to see how you both feel when you are using them. If you are not sure that it's working out, you may want to ask someone else, either instead of or in addition to your main partner. You might find that you want a back-up person, because a long labour can be hard on your partner as well as on yourself. You might even choose to employ someone like an independent midwife or a doula (a professional birth attendant) to give you additional support.

It could be that you want several people there, offering different types of support, or you might decide that you would prefer to be on your own as much as possible.

Think carefully about who you want to be present at the birth. If you are not comfortable with the people who are with you then, including the midwife, that discomfort is going to have a negative effect on your labour. And

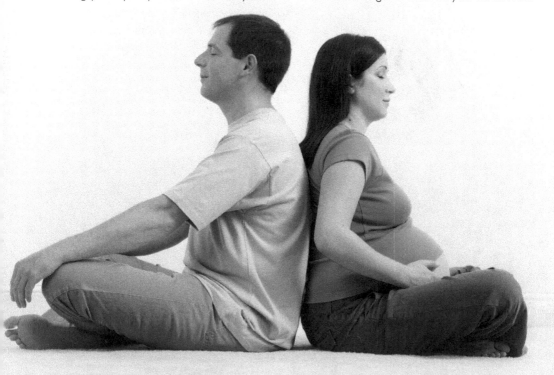

because you may not know how you feel about the people with you until you are in labour, your birth partners must be aware that they might be told to go away.

The role of the birth partner

Traditionally, the partner's role was to keep the birth environment safe. The partner would be the one standing at the door of the hut, making sure no-one unwanted came in. Helping to hold the physical space is still quite a large part of the role, especially if you are in hospital.

Your partner may need to be the one to say that you don't want lots of junior doctors coming in, or to dim the lights so it is not too bright, or to ask people to stop talking. He also needs to be comfortable with questioning medical decisions and finding out if they really are in your best interests, or simply to ask for more time to consider options.

Another thing your birth partner needs to be aware of is that he is probably not going to be thanked during labour for what he does. A birth partner has to assume that if the mother says nothing, then what he is doing is fine. She is not going to say, "Hmmm that feels nice." If the partner's work is effective, then it is enabling the mother to carry on with labour. If it isn't, then the partner has to be prepared to be criticised, told off, maybe even told to go away.

Your birth partner needs to know your wishes and support you in them. If you want to have a beautiful, natural birth, your partner needs to have practised the breathing, physical preparation and touch skills in the book. The book is for your partner as much as for you.

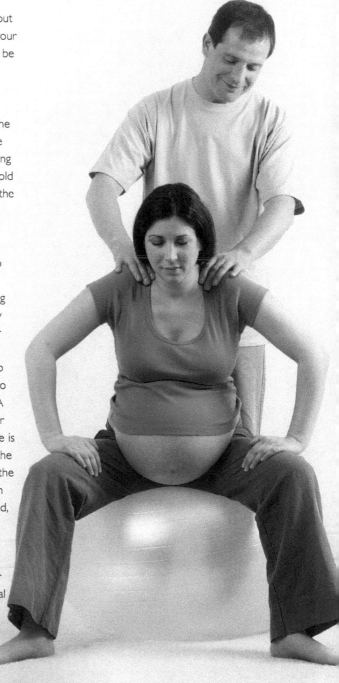

Eating and drinking

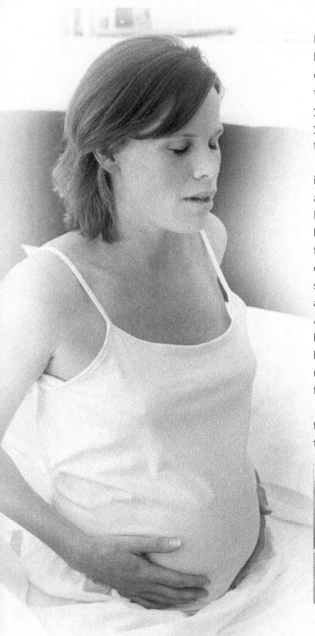

It is important to keep well nourished during labour, especially if it's a long one. Some mothers don't like to eat at all in labour, but if yours is long, then you will probably feel hungry eventually. Until you are in labour, you aren't going to know what you are going to want or need, so have a range of food and drink options available.

If you are giving birth at home, food and drink is not a problem because you can stock up in advance with everything you might possibly need. If you are going to be in hospital, though, you have to think more carefully about the kind of food you may want. You are never going to know exactly what that is until you are actually in labour, so provide yourself with as many different things as you can easily bring so that you have a choice. Also check out what there is available from the hospital canteen, what its opening hours are, and how far away it is from the delivery rooms. It may not always be that practical to go and get food from there.

Don't forget your partner either. You may not feel like eating, but he probably will – especially if the labour is long.

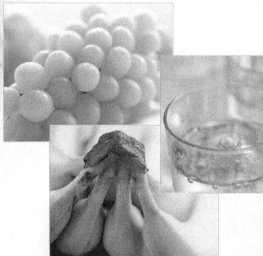

FOOD

Below are some suggestions for you to bear in mind when planning what food to bring in for labour. It is a good idea to choose food that is easy for you to digest, such as a meal of lightly cooked vegetables, than anything too heavy. Go with what you feel like, but make sure you eat something if you are in a long labour, that is, one lasting more than 16 hours.

Fresh fruit such as bananas (although they are mucus-producing they are a good energy source), apples, pears and grapes

Dried fruit, which contains a lot of energy and stores well; dried apricots are also a good source of iron, and figs provide calcium

Salads and raw vegetables are good snacks; have some carrots or cucumber slices to nibble on

Nuts can be hard to digest, but they are very nourishing

Wheat and cheese can be bloating and heavy for many people, but oatcakes and rice cakes are good alternatives

Glucose snacks can help to keep up your energy if you don't feel like eating and labour is prolonged.

DRINK

Water is a great drink to have during labour, either hot or cold, and you can also use it to sponge your face. Fruit juices or smoothies are good drinks for energy as well as for quenching your thirst, and herbal teas can be refreshing, but make sure you have tried them beforehand so that you know whether you like them or not. Avoid ordinary tea, though, as well as coffee and fizzy drinks. Tea and coffee can be too stimulating and fizzy drinks are too bloating.

Preparing your baby

Now to the most important person at the event – your baby. She is just as much a part of the process as you are, and may even be the one who chooses when to start labour off; babies do generally come when they are ready. Just as labour is different for different mothers, so, too, is it different for different babies. Some seem to love staying on in the womb and are reluctant to come into the world, but others can't wait to be born.

It is worth spending a little time focusing on how labour might be from your baby's perspective. You can spend time preparing for labour, but your baby is launched into it. While you are releasing endorphins, your baby is releasing adrenaline. Labour, therefore, is quite stressful for your baby, but it is a stress with which she is designed to cope. In fact, some people believe that labour may be a good preparation for how to deal with stress in life.

Years ago, some psychologists believed that labour was too stressful for babies and they should all be born by Caesarean section. Now they have realised that a C-section is not something babies are naturally designed to go through, and it actually may create more stress than a straightforward vaginal birth. Babies can be helped to process the stress of a C-section, but parents do need to be aware that their babies may need a little extra support to make the adjustment to life outside the womb.

That is not to say that babies can't get over-stressed during a vaginal delivery. There is a fine balance and if the labour is particularly long, or the baby gets stuck, or the cord is wrapped around her neck so that she is not getting

enough blood, then the stress can become too much and is known as "fetal distress" or "compromise". This can be a reason for having to deliver the baby immediately by C-section or forceps. In such situations, it is important to try not to add to the stress that your baby experiences by being stressed yourself. Whatever happens, relaxation must always remain a high priority.

What your baby "knows"

You have to remember that by the time she is ready to be born, a baby is a very aware being – although opinion differs on how aware and when that awareness comes.

By the time of birth, a baby has been aware of touch since week 8, sound since week 22, and light since week 30. It is interesting that touch is the earliest sense that develops. The baby has learned to be aware of feelings of being touched from the inside (by the womb contracting or the movement of the mother's intestines) and also from the outside (through the touch of the mother on her abdomen).

Your baby is also aware, in her own way, of everything that you do. Hormones in the mother do pass through to the baby, so if you feel stressed in labour, you will add to your baby's stress. If, on the other hand, you are relaxed, your baby will be more relaxed.

Keeping in touch

Labour is a complete unknown for your baby, as well as for you. If you have been talking to and massaging your baby during pregnancy, then it is good to continue doing that throughout

Connecting with your womb and baby

This simple relaxation exercise will help you to become attuned to your womb and connect with your baby.

Find a place where you can sit comfortably. Focus on your breathing, and with each out breath allow your breathing to become deeper and your body to feel more relaxed. Close your eyes, if you wish, and focus your mind on your womb. Be aware of your womb as a space; envisage a subtle light within it and be aware of its colour. Breathe gently, resting all your attention in your womb. Sense each breath going to its centre, bringing with it more light. Let each out breath take with it any doubts or anxieties you have about your labour.

Your womb will gradually become free of tension, allowing you to hear your baby. Let your breath go in and out and, as it does, ask your baby to speak to you. For the next few minutes, sit and listen. Your baby will begin to release emotions, thoughts and dreams. You may feel your breathing change. Let go of any fears or anxieties you may have about labour. If negative emotions appear, simply tell yourself that they are leaving you easily and comfortably. If voices of doubt start to surface, gently tell them to leave. As you continue, allow your womb to reveal itself as safe and warm. Once you feel a sense of peace and connection, allow yourself and your baby to be in this relaxed space for as long as you need.

When you are ready to ease out of your relaxation, gradually become aware of the movement of your breath out and in, and of the room around you. Eventually, on an out breath, allow your eyes to open.

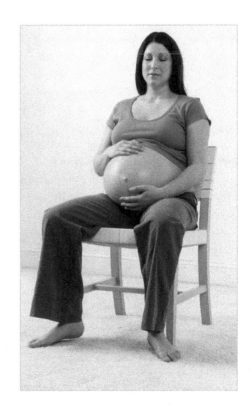

labour, if possible, because it offers your baby reassurance and familiarity.

You or your partner could communicate with your baby by touching or massaging your abdomen. If you played music that made you feel relaxed while you were pregnant, your baby will also have felt relaxed. Playing the same kind of music in labour, and even after the birth, will help both you and your baby to relax.

It is never too late to have a name for your baby while she is in your womb. You can use this name to talk to her while you are pregnant and continue using it in labour. It could be the name that you are intending to call your baby, but it also could be a "womb name". I called my daughter "Little Fishy" and my son "Cherry Berry". Sometimes people worry that such a name might stick, but when you meet your baby, you will find her new name. In our family, the womb names haven't been used since the first few weeks, although we sometimes fondly remember them! However, sometimes womb names feel appropriate and so you may keep on using them.

In the last few weeks of your pregnancy, you can write a journal to your baby about the experience of birth. You can explore what you are going to do to support her during the process of labour. You also can talk to her about this while you are massaging your abdomen (see page 64).

You can continue to communicate with your baby throughout labour. In fact, by cutting off from your baby, you may make labour more difficult for her. You can focus on or even talk to your baby while you are having a contraction. If things do get more difficult, you can talk to your baby about what is happening. Many mothers find focusing on something positive, such as their baby, rather than something negative such as the pain, can really help them have a more positive attitude to the birth.

Readying your baby for birth

This visualization exercise helps your baby to anticipate birth. Please do this only in the last few weeks of your pregnancy, because you don't want to focus your baby on her birth before she is ready, unless you are preparing for a premature labour.

Find a comfortable position in which to relax, either sitting or lying, and close your eyes. Breathe slowly out and in and follow the pattern of your breathing. With each out breath allow your breath to deepen,

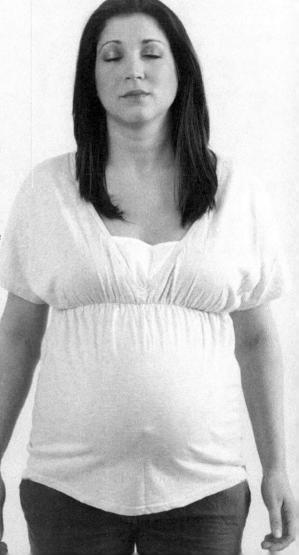

let yourself become more relaxed, feel your abdominal muscles gently drawing in and become more aware of the baby in your womb.

As you breathe out, be aware of how your baby is now – safely growing inside your body, inside your womb's watery environment. Notice whether your baby's body is moving around, or is still. Think how it must be for your baby in your womb, hearing the sound of your heartbeat. Be aware that she never feels cold or hungry and sleeps when she feels like it.

Now tell your baby that she is going to remain physically in this safe space, but you are going to take her on an imaginary journey into the future. She is going to travel outside your body to her new home. You imagine the progress of this journey from her point of view.

The walls of your home are tightening and squeezing your body. You feel squashed and new sensations flood you. Everything seems to slow down for a few moments. Then the tightening gradually subsides and you begin to feel familiarity again – the sound of your mother's beating heart, her voice and other voices around, maybe music and singing which you have heard before. You begin to feel comfortable again and start to relax. Then the uncomfortable feeling of being squashed begins to happen again. You feel as though you are being pushed out, being dragged out of your safe, comfortable space. You are not sure what you are feeling. Maybe there is something new and exciting beyond the walls of your womb world? Maybe there is something scary out there? You are not sure, yet you feel yourself gradually being pushed out. Are you ready for this to happen?

As you are slowly being squeezed out of your home, you feel doubt. Sometimes you get stuck and are unsure whether you can move forward or not. It's like you are going down a long narrow tunnel. Your whole body is being squeezed from all sides.

Eventually, you feel your head being squashed even more but then the pressure starts to ease and you feel some new sensations. Your body starts to twist and turn, and all of a sudden you are in a huge space. You are in another world outside your womb. Is it cold? noisy? bright? Suddenly you are enveloped in warmth, can hear that familiar heartbeat – louder now – and have an overwhelming urge to find nourishment.

After taking your baby on her imaginary journey, slowly begin to focus on your own breathing and become aware of the present moment, with your baby safely inside your womb. Take notice of her in this moment. How is she moving? Is she kicking around or being still? You may even want to talk to her for a few moments and reassure her that the real journey has not yet begun. Be aware of your breathing and follow the movement of your breath as you breathe out and in. Be aware of the way you are sitting or lying and of the space in which you are resting. On an out breath, open your eyes.

Your baby's position

How your baby is positioned in the womb will have an influence on the type of birth you both will have. The best position is for your baby to be head down (cephalic) with his spine facing away from your back (in an anterior position). This means that his head is more tucked into his body so a narrower part of his head comes down the birth canal first. It also means that your baby's back is away from your back.

If your baby's back is against yours (in a posterior position), labour may be painful. It also may be more difficult for your baby's head to come through the birth canal. When a baby is in the posterior position, the first stage of labour contractions "work" to get your baby into a better position. As a result, you may have a much longer and often more painful first stage than if your baby had been in a good position to start with. However, it is perfectly possible to have a beautiful birth with a back-to-back baby.

If your baby is in the bottom-down (breech) position, then it is still possible to have a normal labour although most obstetricians these days are not keen on risking the possible complications and usually advise a Caesarean. If you really want to have a natural birth – especially if this is not your first baby – you will need to find someone who is experienced in delivering breech babies. This may not be easy, because sadly those skills are being lost.

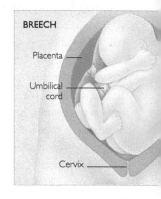

BREECH

Placenta

Umbilical cord

Cervix

If your baby is lying across your uterus (in a transverse or oblique position), then neither his head nor his bottom is down in your pelvis so it is not possible to give birth vaginally unless your baby turns. It is not that uncommon for a baby to be in this position in the last few weeks of pregnancy, especially for a second pregnancy, but usually a baby will turn head down before birth.

Checking your baby's position

To find out what position your baby is in, ask your midwife to help you identify it after 28 weeks. If he is posterior, all his limbs will be at the front of your body, and often you will feel lots of movements and lots of bumps and lumps and spaces. If your baby is anterior, you will feel the hardness of his back and spine to one side of your front and his limbs on the other side. It is hard to feel if your baby is breech, as bottoms feel very much like heads, so you will need your midwife to check this for you.

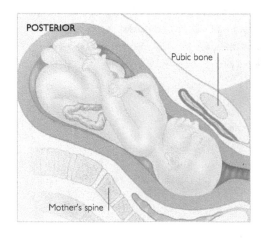

POSTERIOR

Pubic bone

Mother's spine

Achieving the optimal position

You can help to get your baby to get into a good position by adopting good positions yourself in the weeks leading up to labour. As your baby's bottom and back are the heaviest parts of his body, if you lean forward then his back will come forward as well, into the anterior position. You also can help your baby to move deeper down into your pelvis by adopting positions such as the squat. He will be moving deeper down in your pelvis in the last few weeks of pregnancy, and will continue to move deeper down during labour. These exercises, and others to help your baby be in a good position, are covered in detail on pages 26-47. Remember to keep practising them.

HELPING YOUR BABY TO TURN

If your baby is breech, then you need to rest with your bottom higher than your head. This knee-to-chest position works by helping the baby's bottom, which is heavier than his head, to go towards the ground, that is, towards your head. This is essentially the same position as lying on your back with your hips higher than your head (the bridge position), but many mothers find that position less comfortable.

Don't use the squatting positions to help your baby to engage, because that can make his bottom go further down into your pelvis.

It is often helpful to visualize your baby changing position, and to talk to and massage him. Try to understand why your baby may have chosen to be in this position. Maybe he is feeling afraid of being born and of the world outside the womb; the ancient Chinese often talked about a breech baby "clutching at the mother's heart". If that is the case, you need to reassure your baby that you are going to be there to help him adjust to life outside.

There may, however, be a physical reason why your baby is in the breech position; for example, he may have the cord wrapped round his neck. In such cases, he might not turn when you do the exercises. If your baby isn't turning, then do seek more information from your midwife about what is going on. Babies do have their own inner wisdom and it is important not to ignore it.

KNEE-TO-CHEST POSTION

This may help a breech baby to turn and creates space for him to get into a good position. The baby's bottom will tend to move away from the mother's pubic bone and his spine away from the mother's spine.

Meeting the unexpected

No matter how much you prepare for your journey of birth, you can never guarantee that things will go exactly as you would like. It is best to be prepared for any eventuality, even for things you don't really want. All I can say with certainty about birth is that it is unpredictable – you have to be open to the unexpected, whatever that may be.

Even if you need medical intervention, you will still find that the skills you have learned from this book will be of help. If you are having to decide whether you need some drugs to help you, or whether you should carry on or agree to a Caesarean, it is still best to make those decisions from a place of calm and relaxation, as much as that is possible. That way you can make a better decision. Essentially, the skills in

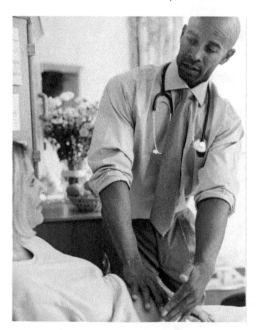

this book are life skills, and you can adapt many of them for use in any situation, especially during the following years as a parent.

When you have gathered all the information and are making your final decision, remember to listen to your body's responses for help with the answer. There will be so much information coming your way from external sources that it is easy to feel bombarded by it. Also, that information isn't always presented in the best way. Bear in mind that even health care professionals are only human, and it is always worth asking for a second opinion if you are not happy with the information you have been given.

The great thing about the skills you have learned here is that their beneficial effects come from within you. You don't have to worry about them interacting with drugs, so you can carry on using whatever you find helpful, whatever the situation. This means that you won't necessarily have to choose between a birth that is totally natural or one that is completely medicalized. You can continue to use the skills, both to reduce the amount of medication you need, and to continue to feel empowered through the process of birth. You then will be less likely to feel that things are being done to you, or that you have lost control. Even if you do end up needing lots of medical support, you can still feel good about the birth, and you will be less likely to suffer from postnatal depression.

USING YOUR SKILLS

Here are a few examples of how you might use or adapt the basic skills to help you if things don't go entirely according to plan. Sometimes you may be just a little too tired and become overwhelmed, but do try to consider the pros and cons of each intervention, and discuss the options with your midwife and your birth partner.

HAVING AN EPIDURAL

An epidural is an anesthetic injection in your lower back, given to relieve the pains of labour. If you opt for an epidural, what you use of your skills will depend on what type you have, and how effective it is. Sometimes epidurals don't offer complete relief, so you may need to continue to work with your breathing while your partner gives you massage.

The massage will probably need to focus more on relieving tension in your neck and shoulders than on your back, and perhaps on gently stroking your legs if they go trembly. If the epidural makes you feel sick or cold, your partner could work on shiatsu points that can help relieve these feelings. The LI4 (see page 83) and HC6 points (three fingers' width down from the wrist crease) are good for the sickness and the HP8 point (see page 74) helps with the cold feelings. Even just holding the cold areas, or wherever you feel needs holding, can be helpful.

As for the positions, you will probably be on a bed but you can still choose the side-lying position rather than lying on your back and you could possibly choose to lean forward, leaning over the back of the bed. Try to continue supporting the natural process of labour as much as you can, because you may well be able to carry on, let the epidural wear off, and deliver your baby yourself, without needing the use of forceps or ventouse.

You may find that you feel quite anxious at this point, especially if pain relief is not complete, but by using the skills you have learned you can help yourself to stay calm and focused.

PETHIDINE AND GAS AND AIR

Having a pethidine injection or "gas and air" for pain relief might make you feel a bit out of it. You can continue to use controlled breathing to help you keep your focus, although with gas and air you may have to adapt the technique as you are having to focus more on the in breath. Make sure that you breathe out deeply too.

Keep your focus on which position is most comfortable, but if you are feeling a little bit out of it your partner will need to give you some extra support. You probably won't want to use the more challenging positions such as the standing squat. You also may find you still want to feel the support of your partner through touch, and indeed, some areas of your body may still feel tense and benefit from massage.

INDUCTION

You can still use your skills if you need to be induced, and you might actually find that you need them even more. Many people assume that if you go for induction then it happens quickly. Often,

Keep including your baby

If things are getting stressful for you, then remember that they also are getting stressful for your baby. You have the doctors and midwives telling you what is going on, but your baby needs someone to tell him what is happening. If you feel that you have lost control and that you are having things done to you, these feelings will be even more intense for him. Touch your abdomen and rub it, and talk to your baby about what is happening, as you would explain it to anyone else. Continue to communicate with him.

however, there is a lot of hanging around and waiting even before you are given anything at all, and when you are in early labour, medical staff are reluctant to give any pain relief because they don't know how long it will take to get labour established.

You will find that using your skills will help you to be more relaxed while waiting, thus helping you be more likely to go into labour. You also can use this time to work on the labour focus points (see page 82) as much as you can, to try to get labour going naturally.

Once you have been started on whatever drugs you are having, you can continue to work the labour focus points. This can mean that you may go into labour having been given just a prostaglandin pessary, or that you have less syntocinon administered than you might otherwise have to have. You are then more likely to have a natural pattern of labour than be forced into very strong, very intense contractions.

When labour starts, you can use whatever you have been practising, as you would with a non-induced birth. You may find that you need to use a lot of it, because an induced birth usually means the contractions are stronger, build to a peak more quickly, and have less space between them.

HAVING A CAESAREAN

Some mothers wonder if there is any point in preparing if they are having a planned Caesarean birth (C-section). The answer is yes. Being as relaxed as you can for your C-section is very helpful, as is having a good connection with your baby.

You may want to think about how to make the C-section as enjoyable an experience as possible for you, your partner and your baby. Even in such a highly medicalized environment, there are often choices you can make, such as bringing in special objects or playing a particular kind of music. You also can use the breathing and visualization techniques to communicate with your baby about the type of birth she is going to have.

You even may find that, depending on the reason for the section, you end up going into labour naturally before it happens, so it is worth being prepared for that eventuality. And, maybe, although this time you have to have a C-section, because of a low-lying placenta or bleeding for example, your next birth could be a vaginal birth. Having prepared for a normal birth this time can help you the next time.

If you require an emergency C-section, it is likely that both you and your baby will become distressed, so try to keep relaxed. Your partner will need to draw upon what he's learned in the book to support both you and your baby. All of the skills you have learned here are essentially life skills, so they are going to be beneficial in some way whatever kind of birth you have. You can use the breathing techniques to help you relax and focus before and during your C-section and afterwards, many mothers have fluid in their lungs and breathing to release the fluid can help. It also is a good idea to practise the exercises, because the fitter you are, the quicker you will recover, and you will be more aware of your body postnatally.

After a C-section, your baby will benefit from some massage because she hasn't had the intense massaging she would have received coming down the birth canal. Of course, you don't want to squeeze your baby in the way she would have been squeezed in labour, but gentle holds and touch may help her make the transition from being in the womb to being outside.

TENS MACHINES

Transcutaneous Electrical Nerve Stimulation machines deliver mild electrical impulses that work in a similar way to shiatsu. Because of this, I usually advise a mother using a TENS machine for pain relief not to have her lower back massaged too much, as that can be overly stimulating. Massage work elsewhere, though, can be done if it feels fine. Use positions with which you feel comfortable and keep using your breathing.

Being aware you may have fears

It is worth noticing if you have any fears around your birth. It is quite natural to have some degree of fear, but some fears may run much deeper and perhaps be related to family patterns, your own birth experience or other traumatic events in your life. If you feel that your level of fear is something more than can simply be released with a breathing or relaxation exercise or talking through with your care giver, partner or friends, then it may be helpful for you to seek out more specific support for releasing this fear, such as with a person trained in trauma therapy, a psychologist or other form of healer.

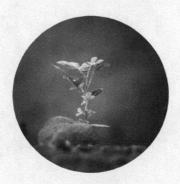

Beyond birth

After the birth of your baby, you can continue using the skills that you learned in preparation for it. They will be very useful to you during the next phase of your journey of parenthood.

Breathing and visualization

Breathing deeply and using the breath to relax will be a great help to you and your partner while you are getting used to the new member of your family. In the early days, you might find you just want to spend time sitting and observing your newborn's breath, but then talking and connecting to her becomes more tangible, and you can repeat some of the sounds and words you used during the pregnancy and birth. Babies are particularly responsive to music and songs, especially those that they often heard while in the womb.

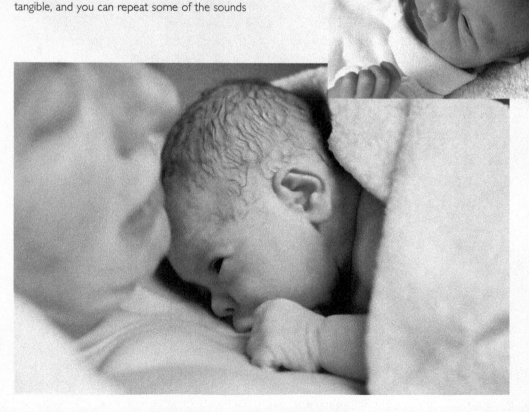

Massage

Continue to massage your baby, and develop your massage routines intuitively as your baby grows. Remember, though, that you may also need massage in these early days, especially to help you cope with sleepless nights and breastfeeding. Your partner will need support, too, so continue to massage each other.

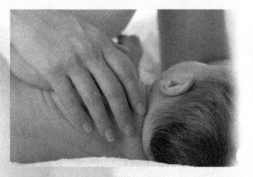

Positions

Continuing to exercise is a great way to help with postnatal recovery, although the birth positions will be too strong to work with in the first few days and usually weeks. You should start with very gentle exercises, but the squatting positions will come in useful later, as your baby gets bigger and you need to have good posture to pick her up.

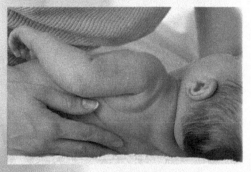

Enjoy

Your baby's new life on earth is just beginning. It is another stage along the birth journey. Enjoy your life as a new mother, and your life as a family.

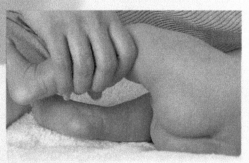

Enjoy your life as a new mother,

and your life as a family

My beautiful birth

QUESTIONS FOR THE MOTHER

Like everything else in life, it helps to plan ahead to ensure that you, your partner and baby experience birth the way you'd like it to be. The following questions can help you to create your ideal birth plan and to assemble the specific tools and techniques to support it.

Note: The mother should reflect on these questions herself. But it can be helpful to go through them together with the partner. It is important that the birth partner knows the mother's wishes and preferences well.

Music and sound
- What kind of music or sounds do I find relaxing in pregnancy?
- How does my baby respond to them?
- Do I think I will want to use these sounds in my labour? If not, what sounds would I like to have during my labour?

Breathing and inner images
- What breathing/visualization seems to work for me?
- Which breathing and images do I think I will use?

Exercises and positions
- Which exercises and positions do I like? Which don't I like?
- What is comfortable for my partner?
- What do I think I will use in labour? Do I think I will use lots of different positions or just one or two?

Shiatsu and massage
- What massage strokes do I like best?
- Which area of my body responded best to being massaged?
- Where do I think I might like to be massaged in labour?

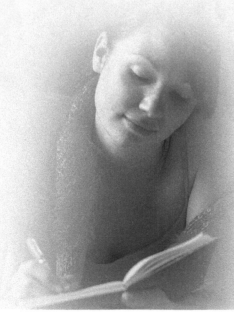

BIRTH PARTNER/S QUESTIONS

- How will I respond to my partner being in pain?
- What kinds of food and drink do I think I will want to have in labour?
- What will I do when I am tired?
- Will I mind not being the centre of attention?
- How would I feel about being asked to go away?
- How would I feel about not being allowed to go away?
- How do I feel about expressing the mother's needs to medical staff and attendants?
- How would I feel asking to change something that the mother is not happy with (e.g. asking people to go away, stop talking)?

QUESTIONS FOR BOTH

- How do I feel that birth is going to be from my baby's perspective?
- Is my baby feeling worried about being born?
- Is my baby looking forward to birth?
- How do I want to greet my baby?
- How are my baby's first few moments after birth going to feel?

How to deal with pain

- How do I respond to pain?
- Both the mother and her partner can think about the last painful experience that they had. Maybe it was physical pain, maybe it was emotional pain. What made it better? What made it worse?

Your birth environment

- What is my ideal birth environment?
- How can I create this environment?
- What are the things I need – heating, lighting, objects, artwork (images or abstract) or photographs, music/quiet (if music, what kind), being home or in hospital, being indoors or outside, use of elements (e.g. do I want to give birth in water, by a fire?)
- What is the key to help me connect with this ideal space? An image, a word, a feeling, an object?

Birth companions

- What kind of person/people do I want at my birth (see birth partners)?
- How many people do I want to have at my birth?
- What sort of qualities will they have?
- What sort of things do I want them to do? Do I want them to massage me, breathe with me, talk to me, get me food, and help keep my environment as I want it?
- Do I want my other children there?

Index

Acknowledgements

Working to support mothers and their partners and babies in supporting birth has been my passion since my own first pregnancy in 1989. I benefited so much from the support of my main shiatsu teacher, Sonia Moriceau, and my partner, Chris Wilkinson, who was also a yoga teacher and homeopath. Chris and I set up Well Mother classes together to share our knowledge and my work has continued to deepen through hundreds of mothers and partners I have worked with over the years.

Since 1997 I have increasingly learnt from the many massage and shiatsu therapists and midwives I have been training with Well Mother.

Most of all I want to thank my two children, Rosa Lia and Bram Delaney, for their support. They have put up with my writing and teaching. A special thanks to Rosa who has edited and given her contributions to the text.

Picture credits:
All original photographs by Jules Selmes
52 Weleda
92–93 Mother & Baby PL/Ruth Jenkinson
21, 107 Photos on Unsplash
  Earth: Sushobhan Badhai
  Fire: Amador Loureiro
  Metal: Wu-Yi
  Water: Zhang Kaiyv
  Wood: Liam Pozz

Illustrations:
Amanda Williams

USEFUL RESOURCES

Well Mother www.wellmother.org
You can use this to access more articles and information. You can also find out local practitioners in your area from the Well Mother register.

Pink Kit www.thepinkkit.com

AIMS: Association for Improvement in Maternity Services www.aims.org.uk
Campaigns for better understanding of the normal birth process and also provides support and information about maternity choices in the UK and Ireland.

Weleda.co.uk

Further reading

- Sheila Kitzinger *Rediscovering Birth* (Pinter & Martin)
- Anne Deans *Your New Pregnancy Bible* (Carroll & Brown)
- Michel Odent *The Scientification of Love* (Free Association Books)
- Pam England and Rob Horowitz *Birthing from Within* (Partera Press)
- Enkin, Keirse Neilson et al *A Guide to Effective Care in Pregnancy and Childbirth* (Oxford University Press)
- Ina May Gaskin *Ina May's Guide to Childbirth* (Vermillion)
- Milli Hill *The Positive Birth Book* (Pinter & Martin)
- Mark Harris *Men, Love & Birth* (Pinter & Martin)

Videos

- Birth into Being: The Russian Water Birth Experience (Elena Tonetti, birthintobeing.com)

Printed in the USA
CPSIA information can be obtained
at www.ICGtesting.com
JSHW060042150824
68134JS00028B/2594

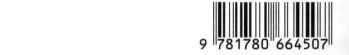

9 781780 664507